There's a lot more to health than not being sick.

Other books by Bruce Larson:

Dare to Live Now
Living on the Growing Edge
No Longer Strangers
The One and Only You
Thirty Days to a New You
Risky Christianity
The Meaning and Mystery of Being Human
Setting Men Free
The Emerging Church
Ask Me to Dance

With Keith Miller:

The Edge of Adventure
Living the Adventure
The Passionate People: Carriers of the Spirit

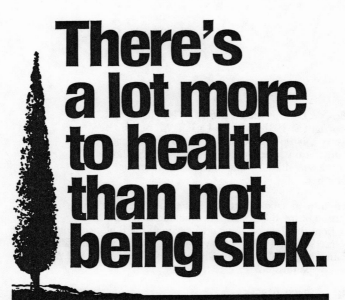

There's a lot more to health than not being sick.

BRUCE LARSON

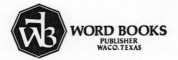 **WORD BOOKS**

PUBLISHER
WACO, TEXAS

Scripture quotations marked KJV are from the King James
Version of the Bible. Scripture quotations marked RSV
are from the Revised Standard Version of the Bible, copyrighted
1946, 1952, © 1971, 1973 by the Division of Christian Education
of the National Council of Churches of Christ in the U.S.A.,
used by permission.

ISBN 0–8499–0288–6
Library of Congress catalog card number: 81–50036
Printed in the United States of America

First Printing June 1981
Second Printing June 1982

To my new family at the
University Presbyterian Church in Seattle
who are helping me live out
the implications
in this book

Contents

Foreword

This book focuses on the mysterious interrelationship between the mind and the body that has fascinated man for centuries. Awareness that feelings and attitudes of the mind can influence the onset and cause of disease in the body dates back to Greek and Roman civilization. Recent research based on modern investigative methods has sparked new interest in this phenomenon and has enhanced our knowledge of this elusive interrelationship.

We have long known, for example, that people who lose a spouse through death have a statistically significant higher incidence of sickness and mortality than others of similar circumstances who have not experienced such loss. Recent studies have shown that the stress caused by bereavement in these individuals impairs their immune system—the natural resistance of the body to infection. These and similar studies have rapidly begun to increase our understanding of how emotional stress contributes to physical illness.

In this book, Bruce Larson describes patterns of behavior and attitudes designed not only to reduce psychological stress but to facilitate wholeness and health. He draws heavily on the wisdom and insights into human nature of the Old and New Testament documents. Though these documents provide no guarantee that the Christian will be free from inner conflict or from outer stressful events, they do provide vast spiritual resources that he can draw upon freely. Mr. Larson's discussion of these resources will prove helpful to every reader.

ARMAND M. NICHOLI, II, M.D.
Harvard Medical School
Massachusetts General Hospital
Department of Psychiatry

Preface

We are entering an extraordinary new age in medicine. Doctors standing at the threshhold of this new age are beckoning us into their research laboratories to show us overwhelming proof of the connection between illness and such things as loneliness, hopelessness, fear, resentment, joylessness, stress, and lack of purpose. In other words, doctors are discovering or rediscovering that people are essentially spiritual. Our feelings about ourselves and others and the quality of our relationships may have more to do with how often we get sick and how soon we get well than our genes, chemistry, diet, or environment.

Clinical observations such as these are on the increase, and they have alarming implications. If our illnesses are caused by things like hopelessness, joylessness, loneliness, and stress, then who is supposed to "treat" us? Doctors are quick to admit that there is little in their medical training to equip them to help patients with these "life problems." Rather, physicians are trained to treat the results of those problems. One doctor lamented to me that he and his colleagues seemed to be practicing "end organ medicine." A problem that begins with a destructive lifestyle or with negative relationships finally affects the body, moving from one system to another until it stops at some particular organ with nowhere else to go. The doctor, pronounces that organ defective and treats it or remove it.

An increasing number of doctors see the fallacy of practicing that kind of medicine and are looking for an alternative. Their own studies indicate that they have no effective treatment for 90 percent of the patients in the average general practitioner's waiting room each week. These people have as yet no medically treatable problems, but they are genuinely ill and may die prematurely.

I hope this book will encourage those dedicated healers who are attempting to practice whole person medicine. But, even more, I hope it will help each of us to be more aware of our own powers to help ourselves and to help one another discover health, wholeness, and the life God intended. The Bible reminds us that Christians are a fellowship of priests, each with the power to be a channel of healing for others. And while the church has largely neglected this important ministry, modern medicine is reminding us that it has never been more urgently needed.

Just today as I was writing this preface, I read a soon-to-be-published article on the subject of hopelessness. The author is Dr. Sanford Cohen, chairman of psychiatry at Boston University's School of Medicine. He claims that a witch doctor actually has the power to kill by means of a hex. Shortly after he points the ritual bone or sticks pins in a wax image, the victim mysteriously dies. Dr. Cohen's explanation is that death occurs because the victim believes in the utter and overwhelming hopelessness of his or her situation. He or she feels trapped, and death is the only escape.

As bizarre as that may seem, Dr. Cohen sees "a striking similarity between westernized man dying from a fear of disease from which there is no escape and the aborigine who dies from an all-powerful spell." A patient sent to a nursing home for terminal cancer can suffer from the same sense of hopelessness. Just as a tribal community rejects a person who has been hexed, says Cohen, so too does a surviving family often turn from the dying member.

Cohen raises the question of self-willed death. This can

happen after a doctor has diagnosed a fatal disease—say, cancer. In voodoo terms, he has pointed the bone. So terrible is the shock that the patient just gives up. The autopsy will show the cancer, but no reason why the patient should have died so soon. Scientists do not understand exactly how this all works, but they do know that a profound feeling of hopelessness causes changes in our norepinephrine levels (norepinephrine is a brain chemical that affects the transmission of sympathetic nerve impulses). So it seems that hopelessness can make us sick even unto death, while hope is a powerful antidote to illness.

The intent of this book is to give you hope about yourself and your physical well-being. It is a book about wellness and wholeness, rather than about illness. It is meant to be a help, a guide, and an encourager for laymen or for those in the healing profession who are eager to explore this new frontier of health. This is also a book for those who are interested in spiritual healing that is both biblically based and clinically sound. My own years of research in this area have convinced me that there is no new medical, psychological, or sociological discovery on the horizon that is not dealt with in the Bible. Basically, we are spiritual beings, and God knew it all the time!

I would like to thank several people who have been of invaluable help in the writing of this book. First of all, there is my wife and life-partner, Hazel, who has been editor, coarchitect, and fellow researcher for all that appears here. My two friends and editors at Word, Floyd Thatcher and Pat Wienandt, have contributed enormously in every way, including love and encouragement. Finally, my faithful friend and secretary, Gretha Osterberg, encouraged me, made helpful suggestions, and typed and retyped this manuscript late at night and into the wee hours of the morning. Beyond these are the loyal friends like Keith Miller, Bill Walker, and Charles Williams, who have stood with me over these past years and who have been a part of the process.

BRUCE LARSON

1.

The beginning of a new era

In a recent survey, the American Medical Association asked several thousand general practitioners across the country, "What percentage of people that you see in a week have needs that you are qualified to treat with your medical skills?" Some replied 25 percent and some 1 percent but the average was 10 percent. In other words, by their estimate, 90 percent of the people who see a general practitioner in an average week have no medically treatable problem. Certainly they are ill and suffering real pain, but their problem is not chemical or physical and defies normal medical procedure. The survey went on to ask what the doctor did for these people. Most of the respondents said they prescribed tranquilizers such as valium. When asked what they would like to do for these people, most of the doctors said they would like to have had time to spend an hour a week talking to these patients about their lives, their families, and their jobs.

Nancy R. is the head nurse in a contagion ward of a large hospital. She has held that job for almost ten years. During that time she has enjoyed perfect health. Three months ago she fell ill. She contracted the same illness that was filling many of the beds in her ward. Talking to a friend after her recovery, her friend remarked, "I knew that job would get you, Nance! That's a dangerous job you have and you'd better give it up."

If Nancy's friend is correct, then it's hard to account for Nancy's perfect health record over the past ten years in spite of contact with deadly germs. Perhaps some other factor was at work. Actually, Nancy confided to me later that a few days before she became ill she discovered that her husband was having an affair, and we talked about it. She came to see a connection between that emotional trauma and the sudden breakdown of her immunity system.

Scientists tell us that when our built-in immunization mechanism is functioning, we can be in contact with deadly germs and experience no ill effects, but when we undergo severe emotional stress, that immunization system shorts out. All of us breathe in germs every day in crowded offices, factories, schools, and public places of all kinds but undue emotional stress can suddenly short out our immunization system.

There's a lot more to health than not being sick

What makes us sick?

Whenever I catch cold, it is inevitably at a time of tiredness and overwork. Does my tiredness and rundown condition make me susceptible to cold germs? Or is my body telling me I need love and sympathy? If I have a cold, my secretary takes pity on me, takes over the office and sends me home. At home my wife fusses over me and sees that I get lots of fluids and TLC. I lie back on my pillows and purr contentedly, even though my nose is running and I have a fever. I feel loved. So we have to conclude that the germ-theory of illness does not entirely explain why we get sick.

Just now we are in a time when more and more people are suggesting that we are sick because of improper diet. We are told, "You are what you eat." My good friend Roger has taken the warning seriously. He reads the label on every product at the supermarket—never touches anything containing preservatives or white sugar. He drinks no coffee. But in spite of all this care, last spring Roger had, without warning, a coronary attack which fortunately was fairly mild. He is still concerned—and rightfully so—about nutrition, but we have to wonder if that is the primary ingredient in good health. It seems ironic that just a few years back the nation's most prominent food nutritionist and originator of the slogan "You Are What You Eat" died prematurely from a disease she had kept carefully hidden from the public.

Jesus lived in a time when all of his neighbors and friends, being good Jews, were very conscious of their diet. But the admonition he gave them is just as appropriate for us today: "Don't you know it's not what you put into your mouth that defiles you, but rather what comes out of your mouth?"

Beyond the physical

Why are we ill? What will make us well? In explaining illness is there a dimension beyond the physical? All of us know people who seem to defy all the laws of health. They are frail,

16

overworked and unconcerned about diet and exercise and yet they stay well and active to a ripe old age. One can't help asking, "Why?"

One answer comes from Victor Frankl, now president of the Austrian Medical Society for Psychotherapy. He concluded that where there is a driving passion or a great purpose in life, the physical body is more likely to survive. When he and a number of other doctors were inmates at Auschwitz during the Second World War, they observed a strange phenomenon in that physically intolerable, life-suffocating camp. Survival did not appear to depend on the health of the inmates. Often the young, the healthy and the strong would die, while the old and frail and sick would survive. Those who did survive had in common a sense of purpose and a hope for the future.

Most of the pioneers and prophets in present-day medicine are coming into a new appreciation for the spiritual nature of men and women. People are not simply chemical and physical substance. The doctor cannot examine the body as a carpenter looks at a board or a plumber looks at a set of pipes. Man is a mystery, an unsolved equation.

Doctor Carl Simonton in Fort Worth, Texas, and his psychologist wife are treating "hopeless" cancer patients with psychological methods and getting startling results. Their techniques include hypnosis, positive mental imagery, and prayer. Their basic assumption is that people have powerful disease-fighting agents resident within their bodies. Rather than relying on outside drugs, medication, and therapy, they help the patient develop an aggressively positive attitude that releases or enhances those healing agents. I would say that they are helping us to discover that faith and hope are big medicine.

A faith universe

Even we Christians (or those of us who profess to be Christians) need to be reminded that we live in a faith universe where the spirit is more real and dynamic than the flesh. So often we have trouble believing the simple facts reported in the Gospel about the Risen Christ. We're told that He walked through walls as though they did not exist; then ate a fish, just as any normal human being would. But these Gospel records are not nearly so incredible if we discard the Newtonian view of the world and adopt twentieth-century physics. Physicists tell us that what appears to be substance is nothing more or less than energy in motion. Even our bodies are mostly space. If you were to remove all the space between the molecules in the human body, a dot barely discernible to the human eye would be left. What appears to be substance is not substance at all. The chair you are sitting on now, your hand itself, or the wall of the room you are in is nothing more than an electronic field that resists penetration.

Medical prophets have long understood the strange spiritual dimensions of faith and healing. Sir William Osler, the dean of North American medicine, was one of the first physicians to unequivocally tie together faith and healing. Just before he died, Osler said this to a group of medical colleagues: "Ladies and gentlemen, I have come to the place where I believe that most of our patients who recover do so because they have faith in the doctor's faith in the cure. The reason we need to find new cures is because we medical people lose faith in the old ones." Is it possible that we get well as much because of our doctor's faith in the efficacy of the medicine as because of the medicine itself?

Sometime ago I read a remarkable story of an early faith healer. Nuñez Cabeza de Vaca, a sixteenth-century Spanish explorer, was the only survivor of a shipwreck in the Gulf of Mexico, and he was washed ashore on the Florida coast. A Gulf Coast tribe of Indians found Nuñez and adopted him. They were a sad lot, victims of drought and famine, and many of them diseased. Nuñez reports that he had nothing to give them, no scientific knowledge and no medicine. All he had was himself and prayer. But to his amazement, in giving them his loving, faithful touch, Nuñez began to see the Indians healed. This is what he said: "Truly it was to our amazement that the ailing said they were well. Being Europeans, we thought we had given away to doctors and priests our ability to heal. But here it was. It was ours after all; we were more than we had thought we were."

This interrelatedness of spirit and body is no longer a new idea. Hans Selye, originally laughed at by the medical world, is now an honored prophet. From his point of view, stress is the number one cause of illness. According to Selye, everybody has stress but how you deal with the stress in your life will determine how well you are and how long you live. Selye's prescription for avoiding stress and maintaining health includes eating sensibly and getting lots of rest and exercise but most of his advice does not sound at all medical. He suggests things like pacing yourself, talking out your troubles, developing an outgoing disposition, *having fun!*

But assuming we could follow Selye's advice and handle the stress creatively, we might still fall victim to another emotion-related illness, according to Dr. James Lynch, medical researcher at Johns Hopkins. In his recent book *The Broken Heart*, he sets forth his absolute conviction that loneliness is the number one physical killer in America today. To prove his convictions he has actuarial tables and graphs based on a decade of research. It is simply a fact, he tells us, that those who live alone—single, widowed, divorced—have premature death rates anywhere from two to ten times higher than do individuals who live with others. He is quick to point out, however, that living alone does not necessarily produce loneliness but the two are often related.

Dr. Lynch's studies show that twice as many white divorced males under age seventy who live alone die from heart disease, lung cancer and stomach cancer. Three times as many men in this category die of hypertension and seven times as many from cirrhosis of the liver. He also points out that, among divorced people, suicide is five times higher and fatal car accidents four times higher. According to his records people who live alone visit physicians more frequently than do married people, and they stay in hospitals twice as long for identical illnesses. It seems the only way many people in our society can find companionship is to get sick.

Nonmedical illness

What can be done to help those who are breaking down physically for emotional and spiritual reasons? In a recent survey, the American Medical Association asked several thousand general practitioners across the country, "What percentage of people that you see in a week have needs that you are qualified to treat with your medical skills?" Some replied 25 percent and some 1 percent but the average was 10 percent. In other words, by their estimate, 90 percent of the people who see a general practitioner in an average week have no medically treatable problem. Certainly they are ill and suffering real pain, but their problem is not chemical or physical and defies normal medical procedure. The survey went on to ask what the doctor did for these people. Most of the respondents said they prescribed tranquilizers such as valium. When asked what they would like to do for these people, most of the doctors said they would like to have had time to spend an hour a week talking to these patients about their lives, their families, and their jobs.

The nature of wellness

Fortunately, more and more people in the helping professions are taking seriously the spiritual nature of people and the interrelatedness of health and emotional well-being. At an international symposium on holistic medicine recently, one of the doctors said to me, "In the past, we doctors treated diseases that happened to be in people. In the future we need to learn how to treat people who happen to have diseases."

In this "whole person" concept of medicine there is just as much emphasis on the nature of wellness as there is on the nature of illness. The medical profession is discovering that health is more than the absence of illness. For centuries doctors have been primarily concerned about pathology. They have focused on the cause, nature and treatment of illness, assuming that the cure of illness would make people well. This study of pathology is obviously still important, and always will be. But assuming that we knew all there was to know about disease, we still would not necessarily be able to make people well. Wellness is more than the absence of illness.

I know a number of doctors who practice with this philosophy. My friend Paul went to see one of them last year. Paul is twenty-five years old. He had never been sick a day in his life. Suddenly, without apparent cause, he suffered great discomfort, upset stomach, diarrhea, frequent headaches. Two or three times a day he experienced measurable fever. He was enervated during the day and sleepless at night.

The doctor he went to see operates out of a well-known clinic. Before his appointment Paul was given a battery of tests at the hands of technical experts. They examined every crack and crevice, tested all his body fluids, X-rayed him from every angle. He took a stress test, a lung capacity test. Nothing was left unexamined.

It was afternoon before he was ushered into the presence of the doctor. After initial introductions, the dialogue, in condensed form, went something like this:

DR. V.: Paul, I've checked out the results of all your tests. I don't see much evidence here that you have anything much wrong with you. But obviously you're having a lot of physical problems. Right?

PAUL: You better believe it. I can't function any more. I simply can't do my job.

DR. V.: Do you mind if we take some time first to talk for awhile?

PAUL: Not at all.

DR. V.: Let's start with some questions. I see you're twenty-five years old. Are you married?

PAUL: No.

DR. V.: Do you have a girl?

PAUL: Well I had one but we broke up about a year ago.

DR. V.: Are you dating?

PAUL: No. There's nobody around that really interests me.

DR. V.: What about your job? Do you like it?

PAUL: Well, I used to like it, but I've been there a couple of years now. I know everything about it and it's becoming pretty dull.

DR. V.: Have you thought of quitting?

PAUL: Actually, I'm looking for a new job, but I haven't found one yet.

DR. V.: Where are you living?

PAUL: I'm sorry you brought that up. When I moved to town I found this great one-room apartment with rent I could afford. It's air-conditioned, and has a built-in washer and dryer. There's a swimming pool, plus tennis courts. It's really perfect. But last fall a friend came to town whom I'd met overseas. He had no place to live and he moved in with me. My old college roommate arrived a few months later and moved in with us. Now there are three of us in my one-room apartment. It's wild.

DR. V.: What about exercise? Do you get some regular exercise?

PAUL: I guess I've been too busy for that lately—I keep meaning to.

DR. V.: How about your diet? What do you eat?

PAUL: I have such a full schedule mostly I eat on the run. My main diet is bologna sandwiches.

DR. V.: Are you a churchgoer?

PAUL: I am a Christian but I haven't found a church that really speaks to my need. The ones I've tried are pretty boring.

DR. V.: You say you are a Christian. Does that mean you take time to pray and read the Bible?

PAUL: Well, no, I haven't been doing that—but wait a minute—
stop! I see it all. You don't need to go on, Dr. V. It's very clear
what my problem is. It's not that there's something wrong with
me; it's just that there's nothing right with me.

Actually, Dr. V. never treated Paul medically for anything but
that interview changed Paul's life. Within a week's time almost
all the distressful symptoms had disappeared. He moved out on
his roommates, applied for a new job, and began dating. He
began to take time for worship, prayer, exercise, play. He paid
more attention to his diet and ate less often at fast-food places.
Dr. V. understood that the practice of medicine is far more than
a matter of chemistry and physiology. Being well is more than
eliminating the negative. Rather, it requires the addition of the
positive.

Paul's story is similar to the one being told by Norman
Cousins, former owner-editor of the *Saturday Review* in his
best-selling book *Anatomy of An Illness as Perceived by the
Patient.* A dozen years ago when Cousins returned from Europe
with a nontreatable illness that left him paralyzed and immova-
ble, he was told by his physicians that his chances for recovery
were one in five hundred. Cousins asked the doctors' permission
to treat his own illness. His first move was out of the hospital and
into a hotel. He reasoned that a hospital was not only full of
germs and expensive but a patient is treated at the convenience
of the staff. Tucked away in his comfortable hotel room, he
began to read up on stress and take massive doses of vitamin C.
He took time to straighten out some of the primary relationships
in his life. Somewhere he had read that laughter was therapeutic, so he decided to program a laugh time for himself everyday.
He sent out for old Marx Brothers movies, and he had his friend
Alan Funt send over old reruns of "Candid Camera." For two
hours out of every day he watched funny movies. The monitor-
ing machines by his bed indicated that after two hours of belly-

laughing all his vital signs improved dramatically. "Ten minutes of belly-laughing gave me an hour of pain-free sleep," he reported. His sedimentation rate came down ten points at a time and, he says, "The more I laughed the better I got." In time his symptoms disappeared, and he returned to work.

It was ten years before Cousins, fearful of giving false hope to others, revealed what had happened to him. Now he is telling the world in his best-selling book and also doing full-time teaching in medical schools around the country. It's exciting to think that our medical people are now asking what wellness looks like.

The need for this emphasis was mentioned long ago by Leo Tolstoy. He says in *Anna Karenina*, "Every unhappy family is unhappy in its own way. But every happy family looks alike." When we are miserable, we have a variety of sources for our misery—for our physical, spiritual, or emotional diseases. Study of one thousand sick gall bladders does not necessarily prepare a specialist for the next one, nor does the study of one thousand depressions prepare a psychiatrist for the next one. It was Tolstoy's view that people who have found happiness have something in common with other people who have also found happiness. The symptoms of health seem to be universal.

Jesus, the most incredible physician of all time, did not focus on pathology. He did not make the healing of diseases his primary ministry. Over the three-year period of his ministry, he healed literally thousands, but there seems to be no indication that He ever went out of His way to look for anyone who was ill. His healing was incidental to his preaching and teaching ministry, to His encounters with people and His concern for their salvation or wholeness.

Jesus had compassion for every sick person. The record indicates no one was ever turned away. But his primary concern was to proclaim the kingdom of God and to become a king of that kingdom. I believe He was demonstrating that if we can find what wholeness or salvation is all about, healing and physical well-being will be a by-product. If we ignore the central message of Jesus' teaching, then sickness will be rampant. To concentrate merely on combatting sickness is counterproductive. There is a better way to help people than to focus on spiritual, physical or psychological pathology.

Making the right choices

In Deuteronomy 30:19, Moses says to the people of Israel, "I call heaven and earth to witness against you this day, that I have set before you life and death, blessing and curse; therefore choose life, that you and your descendants may live."

Do we really have the ability to choose life? For so long in this century we've seen ourselves as helpless victims of the world around us, of everything from germs to genes, environment, heredity and all the forces of life. Now we stand at the beginning of a new era. The old words from God through Moses to his people make new sense. We can choose to be whole people, with God's help. We can choose to be well people. We can't always avoid illness, but we can begin to be and do those things that lead to wellness. We *can* "choose life."

Let's assume that you have a vague feeling that things are simply not right for you. You may even be physically ill. You may be depressed and miserable with lots of known problems, or simply filled with a feeling of unrest and unfulfillment. In these next chapters, I want to talk to you about your health, not in terms of your phsyical problems but in terms of your life problems. I'm going to be asking you questions about seven specific areas of your life. We'll be exploring some attitudes and behaviors that I consider essential to our health and well-being.

Unlike Dr. V.'s patient Paul, who seemed to have nothing right in his life, most of us will find that we have many things right in our lives. If you went to a doctor with a real physical complaint, he would give you the good news that most of you is well. However serious, your illness is caused by the breakdown of just one small part of your body. The doctor would not give you a general body-building course, but would try to find your

There's a lot more to health than not being sick

particular problem and deal with that. As you read these next chapters, I believe you will find you have already chosen life and most of the vital ingredients of wholeness. I predict you will answer yes to most of the questions asked in the following chapters. But let God speak to you then about those one or two areas where you need to make a conscious choice for life—for health—for wholeness.

2.

Is it becoming easier to say "I was wrong"?

The main meeting room was the living room of an old farmhouse. Here people gathered and ate and talked in small groups before the roaring fireplace on cold, Canadian winter nights. But a beautifully framed sign over the fireplace is the thing I remember best. It said, "Do you want to be right or well?"

It's hard to believe that there is any connection between the ability to "be wrong" and admit mistakes, and our physical or emotional health, but this age-old insight is being rediscovered in our time.

Several years ago I visited a halfway house in Western Ontario. It was a marvelous place to send emotionally disturbed people who did not need institutional care, but who simply had lost the power to cope in their own familiar situation. I personally knew a number of defeated, broken people who found new resources and new identity during their stay there.

The main meeting room was the living room of an old farmhouse. Here people gathered and ate and talked in small groups before the roaring fireplace on cold, Canadian winter nights. But a beautifully framed sign over the fireplace is the thing I remember best. It said, "Do you want to be right or well?"

That sign summed up the philosophy of the director and of the whole place. He was convinced that most people who came there had that choice to make. To become well they had to give up the privilege of being right. He felt that the need to justify one's self in the eyes of others was one of the major causes of most mental or emotional illness.

There's a lot more to health than not being sick

Can you answer the question for this chapter, "Is it becoming easier to say, 'I was wrong'?" with a yes? If you can, then that's one indication that you are taking a big step toward being a well person. Maintaining a feeling of rightness is eventually going to take its toll on any of us—mentally, emotionally, and physically.

Most of us would like to think that our penchant for justifying ourselves is simply somewhat neurotic. But it's a fact that in 1980 the terms *neurotic* and *neurosis* officially went out of use in the psychiatric and psychological vocabulary. The authoritative bible of the trade is the *Glossary of Psychiatric Terms*, and this weighty book no longer lists those terms. The professional counselors who used to use the term *neurotic* now prefer to speak of this group of patients as people who have life problems. It seems to me this is a polite term for dumb behavior.

The classic neurotic treated by many psychiatrists and therapists for so long exhibited symptoms of depression, anxiety, sleeplessness, headaches, tension, constipation and a whole host of other problems. Now psychiatrists are suggesting that those symptoms are not the results of any disease of the "nerves," which is what neurosis implies. Rather these symptoms are the side effects of foolish, self-defeating or destructive behavior.

Paying a price for "rightness"

I'm convinced that many of us have an inordinate need to be right and that need is a considerable block to the whole and healthy life God wants to give us. It takes a lot of psychic energy to maintain this constant posture of rightness and eventually our bodies are going to pay the price for the stress that results. Sometimes our fear of being wrong or being caught off base prevents us from any kind of spontaneous, risky living. Martin Luther once said, "Love God and sin boldly." Certainly Luther was against conscious, willful sin in every form. He was not recommending license. Rather, he suggests that to make the avoidance of sin the focus of life is to squander our spiritual inheritance. We are called by Jesus Christ to love God totally, to love our neighbor unconditionally and to love ourselves scandalously. If we do these three things, we are bound to sin by omission and commission. The focus of life is to love God, neighbor, and self, and in doing so you cannot avoid sin.

Do you remember the first time you went to an unchaperoned party with your peers, all by yourself? If you're lucky, you had parents who sent you off with words like, "Hey, I hope you have a wonderful time!" But it's more likely your parents sent you off with injunctions like this: "Be good!" "Be careful." "Come home on time." "Don't hang out with the wrong crowd." "Remember that you are a Larson (or a Christian)." Most of us got some form of parental injunction that implied the main purpose of the evening was to stay out of trouble.

I used to live on an island inhabited by sailors and fishermen. One day I was invited along with a couple of other men to try out a friend's new sailboat. As we began our sail in a brisk breeze in the Gulf of Mexico the owner was at the tiller. He said to the three of us, "You know, I've been sailing for seventy years. Had my first sailboat when I was ten years old. It cost me ten dollars and many hours of repair. I have been sailing ever since, and would you believe that in those years I've never yet tipped over a sailboat?"

The other two men looked at him aghast. "Are you serious?" replied one of them. "You've sailed for seventy years and never tipped over a sailboat? My goodness, you've been careful. I don't think you've ever really sailed."

Those veteran sailors were aware that the fun of sailing is to court the possibility of capsizing. The same principle might apply to our lives. If we're unable to take risks that lead to an occasional mistake, we've been too safe. Maybe we've never really lived.

Nevertheless, none of us wants to be caught off base. Franz Kafka, in his powerful book *The Trial*, tells about a man in a police state who is told that he is going to be brought to trial by the state. He's in a panic. He goes from bureau to bureau, office to office, trying to find out what the charges are. Unable to learn the nature of his offense, he spends his entire life building a defense against any and every possible charge. This story powerfully portrays our universal need to defend ourselves and prove that we are not guilty. Unfortunately, a life built around self-justification is a wasted life.

Perhaps this is the tragedy of ex-President Richard Nixon, one of the most pathetic figures of modern American history. Mr. Nixon was caught in a minor scandal, one which might have been quickly forgotten had he not been so vehement in his defense. His need to "stonewall" wrongdoing so offended the American people that they demanded his ouster from office. Even most of his friends deserted him. What was his primary crime? I think it was not so much that initial wrongdoing as it was his insistence on his own innocence. I believe he is a poignant illustration of the disastrous results of being unable to say, "I was wrong."

The healing climate

Similarly, physical healing can only take place in a climate of openness. Medically speaking, if a person has a wound, he or she has to admit having the wound and allow a doctor to open it up and remove all the foreign particles. Once the infected area is uncovered and treated, healing forces are at work making tissue new again. To deny and cover over the infection courts serious illness and possible death.

This principle is at work as well in psychiatric and psychological healing. The counselor is someone who does not condemn and in whose presence we can lower our defense mechanisms. The counselee can begin to admit to shameful acts and to wrong attitudes and to take responsibility for his or her behavior. It is in this kind of relationship that healing of the mind and spirit begin. Dr. Salvador Minuchin, who practices psychology in Philadelphia, is the originator of family therapy. Minuchin believes that those who are functioning poorly, medically, emotionally and often physically, have not gotten into that state all alone. They have experienced this breakdown within some kind of a group that is supporting and encouraging the illness, if not causing it. He brings the whole family together to treat the particular problem evidenced in one of its members.

One of the commonest contributing factors in physical or emotional illness, according to Dr. Minuchin, is the family who will not allow someone else to be wrong. The patient is often the product of an overprotective family who keeps excusing or apologizing for him or her. Part of therapy is to help these patients free themselves of the very families who are continually supporting and defending them.

Exercising our choices

This inability to permit others to be wrong is affecting our whole penal system, according to two doctors at St. Elizabeth's Hospital in Washington. Psychiatrist Samuel Yochelson and psychologist Stranton Samenow have had sixteen years' experience at a federal mental institution. During that time they have done studies to prove that we are not effective in changing criminals because we simply cannot allow criminals to be wrong. We are lenient toward and sentimental about them because we think that people like that must be "ill." We cannot believe that anyone "in his right mind" would commit such stupid and criminal acts and commit them repeatedly.

These two pioneer doctors can produce voluminous evidence to indicate that criminals freely choose to commit crimes, that they are not mentally ill. Drs. Yochelson and Samenow insist that if we treat the criminal as someone who has consciously chosen destructive and criminal behavior, then he or she can be challenged to choose to behave differently. If we assume that the criminal is ill and therefore not responsible for the act, they believe there is no therapy which will effect a change.

It seems to me these two doctors are speaking about the general "no blame" attitude now permeating all of our thinking with respect to crime and criminals. People of good will want to believe that poverty or mental illness must be the root of most crime. We tend to overlook the fact that many muggers have more money in their pockets than do their victims. Perhaps society's permissive and accepting attitude toward criminals is one of the biggest blocks to demonstrating the kind of tough love that will free criminals from their destructive patterns.

But the words "I was wrong" are difficult to say, whoever we are and whatever our circumstance. I heard James McCord, president of Princeton Theological Seminary, say in a lecture, "To sin is man's condition. To pretend he is not a sinner, that is man's sin." That's the good news—that we're all bad. God seems all too aware of the fact that we are going to make mistakes and even consciously choose destructive behavior. But the message of the Gospel is that God wants us to own up to this, to make restitution, to believe that we are loved and forgiven and to live accordingly. The very heart of sin is to play at innocence. If we really understand the Bible we have to revise our thoughts about heaven and hell. We think hell is for bad people and heaven is for good people. Actually, hell is for people who think they are good and heaven is for those who know how bad they are.

In 1 John 1:9 we read, "If we confess our sins, he is faithful and just, and will forgive us our sins and cleanse us from all unrighteousness. If we say we have not sinned we make God a liar and his word is not in us." But so many Christians and churches seem to communicate the very opposite of that. We hold up a model of Christian life in which a person walks circumspectly and with perfection before God. We have suggested that Christ came to give us a new birth that will return us to some kind of prenatal innocence. This is absolutely contrary to the biblical message. In Jesus Christ, God gives us the gift of responsible guilt. If I own my mistakes and my sins and can say that I and no one else is responsible for them, then I can be forgiven.

I think we have been misled by the translation from the Greek which comes to us in these words, "Be perfect, even as your

Father in heaven is perfect" (Matt. 5:48). The Greek word translated as "perfect" actually means "fulfilled." It means that we're to be the unique creation that God made. A flower is "perfect" by simply being a flower. This kind of perfection has nothing to do with moral perfection. It has to do with fulfilling our unique destiny. But if we interpret that verse to mean moral perfection, then we think when we become Christians we will be sinners emeritus.

According to the Bible, there is no sin we can commit for which we cannot be forgiven except the sin against the Holy Spirit. Now, what exactly does that mean? Well, it seems to me that if we believe in the Atonement for all sin through Jesus Christ, then the unforgivable sin must be to refuse to be forgiven. The Bible tells us that the role of the Holy Spirit is to convict us of sin and that the Holy Spirit will let us know when we have done something bad or unloving or unjust or corrupt. When this happens, we begin to suffer pangs of conscience. If we listen to those pangs and say, "I'm sorry for what I have done," we can change our behavior, claim forgiveness, and move on and be new beings in Christ. But if we deny those pangs and say, "Well, under the circumstances I had no choice," or, "Other people do the same thing and worse," or, "In my position, the rules don't apply to me," (which Mr. Nixon apparently said) then we have sinned against the Holy Spirit and forgiveness is not an option.

To put it another way, let's say I am describing an argument with my wife to a friend. I say, "But all I said was, 'Is your mother coming for a visit again?' And she blew her top." When we preface anything with "All I said was" we are in trouble. Those four words must be among the most destructive (and illness-producing) words in the English language. They imply that I am sane, logical and loving and the other person is an irrational nut. I wish I could promise myself that I would never again use the words "All I said was—"

Aaron, Moses' brother, is a classic example of this kind of self-justification. When he and Moses were in the wilderness, Moses left for a time to climb the mountain to receive the Ten Commandments from God, leaving Aaron in charge. When he finally came down from that momentous encounter with God's set of rules to live by, he found the people of Israel worshiping around a golden calf, an idol to Baal. In a rage, Moses confronted Aaron, "What have you done! How dare you lead God's people in the worship of Baal when God himself has led them out of bondage into a new land?"

Here is my free translation of Aaron's reply: "Now, Moses, don't fly off the handle. Are you going to believe what you see here, or are you going to believe me when I tell you what really happened? You were gone a long time. We were worried and we missed you. In fact, we got deeply depressed, and you know how it goes when you're worried and down. We thought we'd throw a party and forget our problems. We did a little drinking, a little orgying and things got out of hand, the way they do when you're having fun. At the height of this orgy we decided to throw all of our gold jewelry into the fire, and guess what happened: out came this golden calf." Aaron's problem was not his sin against God. God can forgive even idolatry. Aaron's problem was that he had to defend himself. He saw himself as entirely innocent, and that was his undoing.

From the biblical perspective, we do not have any claim to innocence. Our guilt began with Adam, and in the New Testament we find even the Apostle Paul agonizing over his inability to do the good he intends, doing instead those things he does *not* intend to do. If we, like Aaron, do not have the option of insisting on our innocence, what is our stance as Christians in the face of our continued disobedience?

We need to catch again something of the vision that God had when He created us. Romans 8:15 says, "All of Creation is standing on tiptoe to see the sons of God coming into their own." I love that verse and the suggestion that all of the galaxies and all conscious life wherever it is in the universe is watching this little pea-sized planet. Imagine, they are on tiptoe to see what we can become as God's creation. God has never made anything like us ever before. Now, if anyone thinks this means that we're supposed to be perfect, he or she has missed the point. You and I are not perfect. We are disobedient and rebellious part of the time. But we have a great capacity for love as well and that makes us exciting creations.

Is it becoming easier and easier to say, "I was wrong?" When we are free to admit our errors, relationships have a new dimension. Most of us get into trouble because we judge other people by their actions and ourselves by our intentions, and, of course, our intentions are always good. When my wife is hurt or angry because of something I have done, I am immediately on the defensive. I remind her how much I love her and insist I'd never do anything to hurt her. I have a hard time believing I could have done anything unloving when my intentions were so good. How much all of my relationships would improve if I could attribute good intentions to those who hurt me and at the same time hold myself accountable for my actions, no matter how noble my intentions.

I think we would have a positive hold on health and wholeness if we could live our lives by this royal rule. Make excuses for others—they meant well—but not for ourselves. This is the very heart of understanding God's grace.

So much of our inability to say "I was wrong" stems from our need to be successful and to win. But an important part of the good news of God's love for us in Jesus Christ is that we don't *have* to win them all. Most of us think that it proves God is with us when we go from success to success. Actually, most of us will fail more often than we succeed, and the real proof that God is with us is that we no longer have to defend our failures or pretend that we have succeeded. If I'm not defensive about my failures, but own them, God can redeem them and make compost out of them to nourish the soil out of which wisdom and compassion and insight can grow.

3.

**Have you
quit blaming
others
for your
problems?**

I have done a great deal of counseling in my lifetime, both as a friend and as a pastor, and by far the largest number of people who come to see me are those who are in pain because of an unsatisfactory or hurtful relationship. What I hear most of them say is, "If only he or she would love me or love me more or love me differently or more completely or in more fulfilling ways."

Hazel and I were attending a week-long advanced Gestalt workshop the first time I was confronted by the question, "Have you quit blaming others for your problems?" About a dozen of us met for day-long sessions to "work" with a very skillful trainer whose primary goal was to get us to "take responsibility for our lives." Within that group, it was not acceptable to say, "It makes me mad." Our trainer would insist, "No one can make you mad. You choose to allow someone or something to make you mad. You are not someone else's victim." If a group member in great pain cried out, "It hurts," the trainer would respond, "You must say *I* hurt. There is no *it*."

The whole point of the workshop was to help us see that we have autonomy over our lives and our emotions. We are not victims, although certainly there are genuine victims in life—racial, political, economic and sexual victims. Those with serious physical handicaps are victims. Hungry Third World children are victims. The Jews in Nazi Germany were victims. But I am convinced that in the arena of personal relationships there are simply no victims. People hurt us or disappoint us or fail us because we allow them to.

I love the story of the two women who met at a cocktail party after a separation of many years. After the initial delighted exchange of greetings, the first woman noticed that her friend was wearing an extraordinary diamond. She could not help commenting, "That is the most beautiful and enormous diamond I have ever seen." "Yes, it is an unusual diamond," was her friend's reply. "It is the Calahan Diamond. And it comes complete with the Calahan curse."

"What is the Calahan curse?" the first woman wanted to know.

"Mister Calahan!" was the response.

Now Mrs. Calahan understood that she was not a victim; she had committed herself to a life that was going to be difficult, but it included wearing one of the most spectacular diamonds in the world and she had counted the cost. With the ring came Mr. Calahan, and with eyes wide open she bought both. I think that my Gestalt trainer would consider her a healthy person.

This whole idea of "no victims" was rather new to me the summer we took part in the Gestalt workshop. But since that time, the message has been coming through from a number of other sources. That same year, some friends and I hosted a national conference at which one of the speakers was Dr. William Glasser, controversial psychiatrist and author of the book *Reality Therapy*. Glasser's whole talk centered on the idea that healthy people do not make excuses. For example, he said, there is never a good reason to excuse yourself for being late. Let's say you've missed an appointment for any number of what you consider good reasons: traffic was heavy, the subway broke down, the elevator stalled, you took a last-minute phone call. According to Glasser you should have taken all those possibilities into account and allowed sufficient time. The only pertinent excuse for being late is, "I'm sorry, I guess I'm incompetent to run my life." We were challenged to say that the next time we were late. Say that for a week and the chances are you will stop being late. I accepted that challenge and found to my embarrassment that it took just one late appointment to cure me of a lifelong habit. I had been late in the past simply because I wasn't competent. When I stopped making excuses for myself, I discovered I had it in my power to be on time.

Taking responsibility in relationships

I believe we have made a start in choosing health and life if we can begin to take responsibility for the circumstances of our lives. But it is even more essential to take responsibility for what happens to us in our relationships—especially those primary relationships with families, close friends, co-workers. I have done a great deal of counseling in my lifetime, both as a friend and as a pastor, and by far the largest number of people who come to see me are those who are in pain because of an unsatisfactory or hurtful relationship. What I hear most of them say is, "If only he or she would love me or love me more or love me differently or more completely or in more fulfilling ways." Most of our psychic, spiritual, and emotional pain is caused by the breakdown in our primary relationships. And it is precisely in these relationships that we have the power to make choices— healthier choices.

Recently my mother died. She was full of years and a great lady. She loved the Lord with a passion and loved her neighbors of every kind, color, age and economic status. When she was eighty-five she was a volunteer at the Cook County Hospital in Chicago, cutting patients' hair and fingernails, carrying bedpans, writing letters and doing general chores. One day a week she worked in an inner-city thrift shop distributing clothes to the poor. In a program sponsored by her church, she tutored a child from the ghetto and taught her to read. I cannot say enough about my mother's life of service and her genuine caring for people.

But having said all that, I must also say that though my mother told me often that she loved me and demonstrated this in many tangible ways, she never made me feel that I was O.K. I spent a lifetime of carrying home my trophies, large and small, without ever getting an enthusiastic response. Toward the end of her life, we were neighbors geographically, and we had dinner together two or three times a week. I was still saving my goodies for her, hoping to impress her—my new book, an article about me from some newspaper. Invariably she would examine the prize blandly and without much comment. Just as predictably, anger and frustration would well up in me and cause me to withdraw from the conversation or to become somewhat hostile.

Our children, at that time mostly grown, tried to help me. They'd say, "Dad, get off Grandma's back. She's a great person, but she doesn't like herself very much, and since you're part of her she doesn't think you're neat either. Quit playing your life to her! It's a no-win deal."

Now, my mother was embarrassingly extravagant about my children and their accomplishments perhaps because they were only partly her progeny. She was extravagant in praise for my wife, with whom she had no biological connection. But I believe the kids were right: her own sense of no worth extended to me, and I had the power to stop being a victim of her inability to respond the way I wanted her to. My problem was not my mother. My problem was myself. When I stopped giving her the power to make me unhappy or angry, she could no longer hurt me and I could love her and accept the kind of love she was able to give me.

Taking responsibility for our choices

But you do not have to go to a Gestalt workshop or to a psychiatrist to perceive that taking responsibility for your life is an important route to health and life. Abraham Lincoln once said, "Everyone over forty is responsible for his face." If you are constantly angry, anxious or depressed, your face (and I would say your body in general) will reflect that. People who refuse to be victims in relationships can begin to celebrate life with joy and that will be translated into physical health. Lincoln also said, "People are about as happy as they make up their mind to be," which you might consider a variation on the same theme. He is suggesting that we have it in our power to choose happiness. Too often our perverse natures choose the opposite.

Jean Paul Sartre, the existentialist playwright and author, recently deceased, brought a brilliant insight into our plight in his famous short play *No Exit*. In this play, Sartre, an atheist, shows us graphically what hell is. Few Christians could give us a more exquisite picture of that ultimate alienation and separation. The play presents us with three people, a man and two women, locked forever and ever in a room with no doors and no windows. The man is in love with Woman A. But Woman A is a lesbian in love with Woman B. Woman B is straight and in love with the man. Each of these three people is in love with someone who does not return his or her love and there is literally "no exit."

But, of course, there is an exit. Any one of the three could turn around at anytime and choose to love the person who loves him or her and find a relationship of love and intimacy. One dimension of hell, in this world and the next, is to choose an impossible love and to go through eternity with one's love unrequited. We have no control over how other people will feel about us. If I have made up my mind that only the love of a particular person will satisfy me—be it wife, husband, parent, child or friend—I am setting myself up for a real hell. Even God himself cannot make anyone love Him. God, who loves everyone ultimately, says to the person who refuses His love, "Well, have it your way." And the final result is ultimate isolation, alienation, and hell. I don't believe God sends anyone to hell. Rather, hell is a place to which people insist on going. God has given us freedom of choice in every area, including that of relationships. So in my life, if my mother does not love me as I wish she would, I must accept that and find others who will give me the kind of supportive, affirming love that I need. I cannot control others but I can choose the people to whom I direct my love.

The other day a young man I had never met before came into

my office. He was twenty-five years of age, had graduated from a local university, and was now working in Seattle. Arriving unannounced, he still looked the part of the scruffy student with full beard, long hair, and the inevitable bib overalls. He confided his loneliness and described the past few years of his life, which revolved around a rather menial job and lots of drinking, drugs, and sex. His friends embraced the same lifestyle. But he was bored and empty and desperate to be rid of all these destructive habits.

I was immediately aware that he really meant business, because in no sense at all did he blame his friends for his lifestyle. He took full responsibility for his past life. He said he wanted to find God and to find a friend. This young man made a promise to God that day to begin a new life and he has. But I don't think that would have been possible if he had blamed his companions or his circumstances. He realized he was free to choose a different way to live and that's what he did.

No helpless victims

Sometimes we hang onto the role of innocent victim because we have been told all our lives to "grin and bear it." Unfortunately we were told too often to "grin and bear" situations we had the ability to change. When we fail to take responsibility to change those things that we can change, life may break down physically and emotionally. To "take arms against a sea of troubles and by opposing end them," or at least some of them, is to choose life and health. Medical people used to speak of a classic cancer type, "the quiet, accepting, make-no-waves" person. I think they've since decided there is more than one cancer type, but the message is still there. To say, "That's the way it is; make the best of it," is not always the healthy course.

Carl Rogers, one of the most innovative psychologists in this half of the twentieth century and the father of nondirective counseling, said recently that he considers only one kind of counselee relatively hopeless: that person who blames other people for his or her problems. If you can own the mess you're in, he says, there is hope for you and help available. As long as you blame others, you will be a victim for the rest of your life. Rogers represents the new revolution in present-day psychotherapy. Too often in the past, psychoanalysis reinforced the counselee's sense of helplessness. Freud gave us some brilliant insights, but many of his theories tend to reinforce our "helpless victim" attitude. In a scathing attack on old-style psychoanalysis, Fritz Perls, a controversial psychologist and founder of Gestalt therapy, said, "Psychoanalysis is a disease masquerading as a cure." He meant that psychoanalysis suggests that you are the victim of what your parents have done to you in the early years and all you can do is to make an adjustment to that. You are locked into your old patterns. Erik Erikson, Freud's most brilliant disciple in our day, emphasized that we can instead transcend our childhood to a very large extent. We have the power to choose who we will be and what we will be.

The will to be well

I had a visit recently with a psychiatrist who was doing a book for his denomination on stress and the clergy. After he had asked me some questions in connection with his book, I asked him one. "Do you ever ask the people who come to see you whether they want to be well?"

"It's strange that you should ask that," was his reply. "Just the other day a severely depressed woman came to see me for the first time. At the end of the hour she asked me if I thought she would ever get better and get over her depression. I thought a minute and said, 'Well, I believe you *can* get better.' I did not have the courage to ask the question you are raising. But I really wanted to say, 'You will get better if you *want* to get better.'"

A friend of mine has had crippling bouts with depression and has been hospitalized frequently in the past for long stretches of time. The last time I saw him, he had not been troubled for several years. Apparently he is cured—as much as any of us can claim a permanent cure. In explaining his recovery, he told me that he had simply come to a point where he decided that he was not going to be depressed any longer. Most psychiatrists, psychologists, and therapists know they are working with many conflicting factors in the patient, not the least of which is the will. In fact it has been such a neglected dimension of therapy that someone has called the will the Cinderella of modern psychology. The client must decide that he or she *will* get well. The question is how to motivate the client to will to get well.

A few years ago in South Florida, where I lived, a neurosurgeon was drummed out of the corps by his medical brothers and sisters. Literally hundreds of his patients had been diagnosed as having some rare kind of encephalitis. His colleagues became suspicious of him. They first denied him group malpractice insurance and then refused him access to the local hospitals. Ultimately he was forced to leave town, but only after a long investigation by authorities both from the Harvard Medical School and the Federal Disease Control Center in Atlanta.

Oddly enough, for months and months afterward, irate and indignant former patients wrote letters to the local newspaper defending this man and decrying the way he had been treated. He was, by their own report, "the best doctor I ever had." These letters really puzzled me. Some time later I happened to meet the woman who had been his head nurse, and I asked her about these fiercely loyal letters. "Oh," she said, "don't you understand? So many of his patients had been told by other doctors that there was really nothing wrong with them. Doctor M. took them seriously. He gave their illness a name and prescribed some treatment. They had at last found a doctor who 'understood them.'" Her explanation made great sense to me. If you want to be a victim, medically speaking, you've got to have some corroboration and cooperation. An honest doctor will tell you there is nothing wrong with you. You must find someone who will enter into conspiracy with you, tell you that you are ill, and treat you.

The Bible, the ultimate source of wisdom about both God and man, points up for us this basic need to blame others for our problems. Adam and Eve are of course the first classic victims. They are in trouble because they have disobeyed God. They have done the one thing God has told them not to do and He holds them accountable. What do they say? Adam says, "It wasn't my fault. It was *that* woman [he doesn't even call her Eve]. She made me eat the fruit." He is innocent, a helpless victim. And what is Eve's explanation? "It wasn't my fault," says Eve. "It was the snake. He made me eat the fruit." The poor snake, having no one to blame, has been cursed ever since, crawling through life on his belly.

The price of wellness

Sin is theological shorthand for man's basic problem—his separation and his alienation from God, nature, himself and his neighbors—and that sin is the direct result of our attempt to blame others for our willful disobedience. This problem is nowhere more clearly illuminated than in Jesus' brief encounter with the man who was lying by the pool of Bethesda, the Jewish Lourdes of its day. The legend was that occasionally an angel troubled the water and the first one in after that mysterious happening would be healed. The man had been there for thirty-eight years, we read, when Jesus walked by and said to him, "Do you want to be healed?" The man's reply goes something like this (again, the free Larson translation). "Do I want to be healed? Are you crazy? Would I be lying for thirty-eight years in this place of healing if I didn't? You must be new here. You don't understand the problem. You see, for thirty-eight years, I have been relying on some people to get me to the pool when the waters are troubled and they never get here on time. For thirty-eight years I have been a victim of their selfishness, insensitivity, and tardiness. Have you ever heard a sadder story? Ain't it awful!"

Now the Bible reports in shorthand and we don't really know all the dialogue between Jesus and this invalid. But I'd like to think Jesus said something like this. "I have a hard time believing that. You look like a clever person. If you wanted to be well, you could long ago have rigged up some clever Rube Goldberg device, the kind that makes the dog chase the cat who hits the paddle which knocks the lever that trips your bed into the pool. Don't blame other people for your problems. I have the power to make you well. But I'm not going to use that until you, by an exercise of will, decide you want to be well. Now think it over. If you get well you'll have to begin to work for a living. You can't lie here by the pool and exchange gossip all day. You can't use your illness to get your way at home. You won't get special attention. There's a price to being well. Do you want to pay it?" The man eventually said yes, because the Bible tells us Jesus said, "Get up and walk. Take your bed with you because you are well now."

In this particular story it seems to me that Jesus is emphasizing the role of the will in physical healing. The story of Lazarus, on the other hand, is quite a different one. Lazarus had been dead three days. His sisters complained that he was beginning to smell. The very flesh on his bones was rotting. But Lazarus was not asked if he wanted to come forth. It was beyond Lazarus' power to respond to any such question. Jesus shouts, "Lazarus, come forth!" And the dead man was raised. The man by the pool had autonomy and Jesus respected that. He could choose wellness and in doing so he found all of the forces of God on his side.

I've had a special understanding of the man by the pool at Bethesda since a skiing accident three years ago in which I broke my leg. For two months I continued my full speaking schedule around the country, wearing a large cast on my leg. At first I feared that traveling would be a terrible ordeal. Far from it. I found I automatically got everyone's attention. Little old ladies helped me across the street and children shared their candy. The airline personnel would drive me to connecting flights as I changed planes in airports. But the best part of all was that in terms of my many speeches, lectures and workshops, I couldn't fail. Even if I bombed, people reacted something like, "Well, it may not have been much of a speech, but what a marvelous man of God he must be to travel all the way out here in that condition and to stand up there on his broken leg to talk to us." I found that, in one sense, when you are ill you can't lose. Even if you do poorly, people admire your perseverance and determination.

I love the television commercial that shows Grandma coming down to fix breakfast every morning even though she is badly crippled by arthritis. We are not told what kind of a cook Grandma is. It's possible that every morning she burns the toast and ruins the eggs. It doesn't matter. This sick lady is going down to fix breakfast and she is a heroine just by virtue of her sacrificial effort. It appears that one reason it takes courage to be well is the edge in life sick people seem to have.

Making hard choices

Jesus refused to be manipulated by sick people though he healed thousands. We are told that he often moved on quickly to avoid the demands of those who might still come for healing. He could not be manipulated, even by his mother (Mark 3:31–35). In the middle of one of his sermons to a large crowd his mother arrived at the door with his brothers and sent in a note asking him to come home with her at once. He is a source of embarrassment and she is hoping he will quit this nonsense. She is really saying, "Why can't you be a nice polite Jewish boy? Come home, work in the carpenter shop, go to the synagogue, eat your soup, be nice to your mother and quit making a spectacle of yourself."

What is Jesus' response? One of God's commandments is that we honor our parents. When his mother confronted him with her wishes for his life, He could have given in and become a victim of her plans for Him. But that would have interrupted what He considered to be God's will for his life and He would have been resentful. Instead, by choosing to disobey His mother He was able to love her and honor her, which He did to the very end. His very last words before His death on the Cross were of concern for her and her future.

What Jesus said to the crowd after refusing to go home with

His mother is the crux of all we are thinking about in this chapter. He said, "Who are my brothers and my mother? Those here who do the will of my Father are my mother and my brothers." At that point in His messianic ministry Jesus did not have the kind of mother who could understand and support him. He could have complained about that and lamented her insensitivity. Instead, He chose to love His mother as she was without having to follow her agenda. He did not try to change her nor allow her to change Him. He turned from her to the crowd at hand and said, "Right here are people who can be my mother and my brothers and who can love and support me in a way that my blood mother and brothers cannot, at least just now."

It's been said that the hardness of God is kinder than the softness of men. Sometimes the best support we can give is to help people make hard choices that lead to life. When people are suffering in hurtful or destructive relationships, we need to do more than say, "Ain't it awful. Aren't you brave to put up with all this?" We can all use help in taking responsibility for our lives and for changing those things we can change.

To cease being victims in our relationships we have to use the power we have. In his book *The Strong and the Weak*, Dr. Paul Tournier, Swiss physician and counselor and author of numerous books dealing with the mystery of life, points out that there are not two kinds of people, the strong and the weak. Everybody has power, he says; we just choose to wield it differently. Each of us has a strategy for getting our way whether we are passive or aggressive, loud or quiet, sulkers or bullies. If you're in a bad relationship with someone else, remember that you have chosen this relationship and you have the power to unchoose it.

Healthy decisions

I saw a doctor recently for a general checkup. I went through all the preliminary tests and eventually saw the great man. He checked me out further, made a few comments about my high cholesterol level, and finally pronounced me a fairly healthy middle-aged man. Now throughout this interview, I was braced to have him tell me I was overweight. I noticed his own inch-of-pinch around the waist and felt that would excuse me from taking any advice he had to give me. (I'm one of those people who hate being told what they must do. Tell me to love God, my country or my family and I'll find good reasons not to. I am negatively suggestible.)

Well, my doctor was prepared for me. He finally took off his glasses and looked at me across his desk. "Tell me, Mr. Larson, how do you feel about your weight?" he asked. How did *I* feel about my weight? What a ridiculous question! *He* was supposed to tell *me* what I should weigh. I looked baffled, so he continued. "Tell me what you would like to weigh." Well, he had me. I thought a minute and mumbled something about wanting to lose ten pounds. "Excellent," he said. "I'd like to help you with your problem. I've got some suggestions for you."

I should add that I immediately bought a bicycle and began to exercise and to watch my diet. My doctor was smart enough to know that if he had made my weight *his* problem I would resist him all the way. Since my weight was really my problem I had no choice but to take responsibility for my life.

Do you really believe that what's wrong with you is not what somebody else is doing or not doing to you right now? One couple I know had been married for over twenty years. At the time of their marriage the wife stated flatly that she would stand for no messing around. For twenty years they lived by those rules, but last year the husband confessed to an affair. It was a mistake and he was sorry about it. He still loved her with all his heart. Could she forgive him? She insisted that she could not. He knew the rules and he had broken them. That's just the way she was. In despair, the man said, "Well, then I guess a divorce is the only course." "No divorce!" she said. "I don't believe in divorce." She would not have him as a husband and she would not give him up as a husband. That's an untenable position and an unhealthy one. As the months went by she began to be discernibly ill. Eventually some friends helped her see that she had to choose. She could choose to forgive her husband and take him back and maybe have the best years of their lives ahead. Or she had every right to divorce her husband and get on with her life constructively. To live in limbo in that relationship, the victim of her husband's infidelity for the rest of her life, was doing harm to herself and her own health.

Or, there's the young father I know who wants very much to be a super dad to his two kids. He grew up in a poor home but he had a wonderful father who was his friend and who spent a lot of time with him, teaching him to fish and to play ball. When this young man married he decided he was going to be the kind of dad to his kids that his father had been to him. But having had a deprived background, he also had a need to be a success in the business world and to give his kids all the privileges he had missed. The day came when those goals collided. A successful executive in a large firm, he has been asked to work evenings and weekends with the promise of a promotion to executive vice-president. Obviously, he has to make a choice. He can have financial success or he can have lots of time with his children. He can't do both or he will probably die of a coronary at age forty. Friends have to help him see there is no one right choice. If he devotes himself to his job, his kids will probably understand and manage just fine. They'll make the most of the little time they have with him. If he drops out of the running for the big promotion, his family will manage on less income and less status. The point is, he is not a victim of his business pressures or of his children's demands. He has freedom to choose and to take responsibility for the direction of his life.

If I am sick because of what other people are doing to me I can change that. I can't choose what my boss does to me, but I can choose not to work for him. I can't choose how my mother and father and brothers and sisters feel about me but if they really do not make me feel good about myself, I can choose to spend less time with them, so that I might love them more. On the other hand, if I have a terrific family I can choose to spend more time

54

with them and reinforce the positive feelings they produce in me. If I am married to someone I love who has a need to put me down all the time, I don't have to believe what that person says. I can love and honor him or her and yet seek for some friends who will give me the affirmation and love that my spouse is presently unable to give. If my only feedback about myself comes from a negative spouse, who may be emotionally crippled, I am handicapped.

A wonderful cartoon some years ago pictured two frogs sitting on a lily pad conversing. One is saying to the other, "You know, I tried that Prince bit for awhile. But frankly, I missed eating flies." If I am in a series of relationships that are simply no fun and which are destroying me, I'm eating flies. God will let us eat as many as we want. When we've had enough, we can choose to quit. We can take responsibility for our lives and become the Princes or Princesses we were meant to be.

4.

How are you fixed for friends?

"Shared joy is a double joy. Shared sorrow is half a sorrow."

—An old Swedish proverb

The question "How are you fixed for friends?" could be phrased in more psychological or spiritual terms. You could ask, "Is there a group of people to which you really belong?" or, "Are there people who know you totally, warts and all?" or, "Do you need to account for yourself, your time to anyone else?" The point is that it is hard to be a whole person without at least a few friends with whom you are free to be yourself, to whom you are accountable. To know and to be known is a vital ingredient for physical and spiritual wholeness.

People who need people

It is a medical, psychological, and spiritual fact that people who need people (and who know it) are the luckiest people in the world. I suppose this is why the human race has historically lived in tribes and then in villages. Those are still the normal living patterns for most of the peoples of the world. Perhaps many of the psychological and physiological problems we see in our American life today stem from our pioneer mentality which was so contrary to this ancient grouping pattern. The Europeans who came here to settle North America found it vast and unexplored. "Self-reliant" was the watchword, and the scout, the mountain man or the pioneer, with his axe and rifle over his shoulder, became the national hero.

In those early days the government gave away quarter sections of land to anyone who would homestead, in order to encourage settlement. People flocked west from crowded cities and villages to have their own land at last. Before they could farm the land they had chosen, their first job was to build a sod hut to live in, and we know that most families built them right smack-dab in the middle of their quarter section. The reason was obvious. People who had never owned land before had a new sense of pride and ownership. They wanted to feel that everything they saw belonged to them.

But that custom changed very quickly. This chosen isolation did strange things to people. Occasionally, photographers went out to record life on the frontier and returned with photographs of weird men, wild-eyed women, and haunted-looking children. Before long most of these families learned to move their houses to one corner of their property in order to live in proximity with three other families who also lived on the corners of their property. Four families living together, sharing life and death, joy and sorrow, abundance and want, had a good chance of making it.

As a boy I grew up in a sort of Swedish ghetto in Chicago where I learned an old Swedish proverb: "Shared joy is a double joy. Shared sorrow is half a sorrow." People of any ethnic background recognize the truth of that. Joy shared with someone is heightened and sorrow is somehow diminished and more bearable.

A psychiatrist in Maryland told me a few years ago that there was an enormous hunger for this kind of shared life among young people in the '60s and '70s. He spoke about the retribalization of America. Almost unconsciously, young people wanted to become a part of a community again, to be held accountable, to know and be known.

Author Jess Lair, in his first book, *I Ain't Much, Baby, But I'm All I've Got*, talks about the salubrious results of spending time with people whom you like and who turn you on. He laments that so many of us, out of guilt, spend time with difficult people whom it is very hard to like. While he does not minimize the need for caring for all sorts of people from time to time, he suggests that we plan to see the people who mean most to us several times a week informally. Many of our mental and emotional dependency problems would be solved, he predicts. What seems to be a selfish drive is actually a survival habit.

Improving behavior

Present-day medicine and psychology are underscoring the therapeutic dimensions of belonging. Behavioral sciences in recent years have expounded the simple truth that "behavior that is observed changes." People who are accountable by their own choice to a group of friends, to a therapy group, to a psychiatrist or a pastoral counselor, to a study group or prayer group, are people who are serious about changing their behavior, and they are finding that change is possible.

Studies done in factories have proven that both quality and quantity of work increase when the employees know that they are being observed. If only God knows what I am doing, since I know He won't tell, I tend to make all kinds of excuses for myself. But if I must report to another or a group of others, I begin to monitor my behavior. If someone is keeping an eye on me, my behavior improves.

For over fifty years now, Alcoholics Anonymous has been helping people find and use the love and power of God to overcome an alcoholic dependency. Certainly a large part of the effectiveness of this group comes out of their appreciation for accountability, community, and belonging. In the early decades of this century there was virtually no hope for the hard-core alcoholic. Medicine, psychiatry and the church had failed the problem drinker. Alcoholics Anonymous has been a model for all kinds of self-help groups. But all of them are based on the miracle of belonging and accountability.

There's a lot more to health than not being sick

A universal fear

But community is more than a resource for overcoming problems. We cannot be whole, fulfilled and fully alive apart from some deep and meaningful relationships with others. Our need for this kind of community is basic. Psychologists tell us that the most primal fear in all people is the fear of abandonment. It's easy to understand why. We come into the world as helpless infants, dependent on adults to feed us, clean us and care for us and most of all, to give us love and intimacy. What infant has not spent countless hours and hours crying out, fearful that no one will come? Whether we are cold, wet, hungry, or simply lonely, we want to know that someone will respond.

Psychologists tell us that this early fear never leaves us and can cause much of our bizarre behavior at either end of the relational spectrum. The gregarious flesh peddler and the hostile hermit may both be motivated by an ultimate fear of abandonment. How much we all need to know that there are people around us who know us just as we are and who love us and who are not only committed to staying with us but who care for us enough to make each of us accountable. One can hardly be whole without that kind of relationship with two or three people.

Life in community

But all that we are learning about community from the behavioral sciences is nothing new after all. If we read nothing but the Bible we would still be confronted with our need for community. I'm reminded again that things are not true because they're in the Bible; they're in the Bible because they are true. If we are truly God's creation and if He is the author of the Bible, then all the new discoveries about man through whatever discipline ought to have their taproots in what God has already revealed to us in the Bible.

To me, there is a guideline for community in Jesus' statement, "Where two or three are gathered together in my name, there am I in the midst of them." I don't happen to think this means that the Risen Christ has promised to be quantitatively more present with two or three people than with one—or that He is present in a special way. But I am convinced He means that if I choose to live out my Christian life alone, there are great limitations to what God can say or do or be in my life. My heart is devious and deceitful and very untrustworthy. I tell myself lies or choose not to know the truth at all.

But if I have chosen to be accountable to a few people, to meet with them and to talk about life as I see God unfolding it to me, then God has a chance to hold up a mirror and show me who I am.

The way we treat one another in our relationships in this life has eternal consequences. Jesus says to believers that whatever we bind on earth shall be bound in heaven and whatever we loose on earth shall be loosed in heaven. There is nothing mysterious about binding and loosing. Everyone knows what it is to be bound up by a fear, an attitude, or a resentment. We are bound, or immobilized, by destructive habits, inferiority feelings, false guilt, or a host of things such as prejudice or self-righteousness. Jesus is suggesting that we have the power to loose and unbind one another in an intimate relationship by our love and sharing, vulnerability, and prayer.

This is one of the awesome and frightening dimensions of the priesthood of believers. Is that the kind of commission you want to have? I don't. Think of the people that you see every week, both in and out of the church. Do you really believe that if you do not love them enough you are binding them forever? This is a frightening challenge. We are given enormous power to use with one another. These binding and loosing powers are seen most powerfully in our relationships with those with whom we're committed in community. I need my brothers and sisters to free me from my bondage. I also need to take responsibility for freeing others.

The Bible also tells us that Christians are to walk in the light.

There's a lot more to health than not being sick

This implies a kind of transparent life in which I do not hide my faults, sins, and shortcomings. When I do not walk in the light, my natural instinct is to cover up and pretend that I am better than I am. We don't need a psychologist or a psychiatrist to tell us what a dangerous lifestyle that is. We walk in the light so we can be the kind of people who can walk away from destructive behaviors. Transformation is possible when I stop spending my psychic energy pretending that something bad is not bad. Then I can spend my energies on those things that are constructive and positive.

The ultimate Model

It seems to me Jesus made a clarion call for community when He said, "Love one another as I have loved you." How did He love us? He became totally vulnerable, which culminated in His crucifixion and death. He did not protect Himself from us. He allowed us to laugh at Him, to mock Him, to spit upon Him, to humiliate Him, and finally to kill Him. He had the power to prevent it but chose not to. And this is the kind of love that He commands us to have one for another.

What does that mean for me? It means that I need to find some brothers and sisters to whom I will give bit by bit the power to hurt me. They will know my secrets—my hiding places—my soft spots—and even my hopes and dreams. This is what friendship is all about, or life in community.

Dealing with loneliness

Jesus also helps us deal with our fear of abandonment, our loneliness. Since Jesus became totally human, He had all of our needs and pains. He too experienced loneliness. His loneliness is seen most dramatically on the night before His trial and crucifixion. In the 26th chapter of Matthew we read that Jesus was overwhelmed by the possibility He had chosen the wrong path as the Messiah, that the Cross was never really God's intention for Him. But, even if the Cross *is* God's will for Him, He is uncertain that He has the courage to go through this most horrible of all deaths. It seems to me that this is the essence of loneliness. Loneliness is not being alone. Loneliness is the fear that you've blown it and that you've fallen short of all the great purposes of your life. In His loneliness Jesus came to three of His disciples, Peter, James and John, and asked them to keep Him company while He prayed through this agonizing time. The sharing of that loneliness with three other people gives us the model for true community. Community does not necessarily remove loneliness but our loneliness can become the basis for our community. As two or three lonely people begin to share their loneliness, they find that they are in a community of love and belonging and acceptance.

Recently I moved to a new town and very shortly thereafter got an invitation to lunch with three other men. They were all strangers to me at that time. Two of the men thought it would be a good idea for the four of us to begin to meet as a small group on a regular basis.

One of the men proposing the group continually avoided my glance, rarely talked to me, cut me off when I did talk, and generally acted as though I were not present. Finally I had a chance to respond to the small group proposal and I said I was going to be very careful about any group I joined. And, pointing to the man whom we'll call Jack, I said, "Jack, I don't want to be in a group with you because you make me feel ignored and minimized and put down."

Needless to say, this straight talk produced an embarrassed silence. Finally Jack said, "Thank you for being straight-arrow with me. You're right. For some reason I took an instant dislike to you." From there he went on to tell us, and me in particular, how lonely he's been in the last two years in his new job. There were tears in his eyes as he spoke of his own inner pain.

I reached across the table and took his hand and told him that what he had shared really made me feel close to him, that I wanted to be his brother and that maybe we were even supposed to be in a group together. This is the power of shared loneliness that Jesus modeled for us, and it changed the climate for that group of men.

Finding a friend

But this kind of community is scary. We all like to make it alone, without anyone's help. Certainly this was true of me for many years. I said yes to God in a bombed-out building in postwar Europe and the whole focus and perspective of my life changed. Jesus became the center and is to this day. But there followed years of powerlessness and ineffectiveness in living as a Christian. I knew Jesus had commanded us to "love one another as I have loved you." I felt God wanted me to find someone with whom I could be as open as I had been with Him—to tell somebody all that I knew about myself and to trust myself to another person. One day, I remember the Lord asking me when I would finally make this next step. I said to Him, "Lord, it's because I can't find anybody who's good enough. If I could find somebody who would not fail me, would not laugh at me, would be my friend even after he knew the worst, who would not gossip about me—I would trust him with the secrets of my life. But all I can find are people like me—shallow, natural-born gossips, and very untrustworthy."

At that point the Lord seemed to say, "Bruce, that's just the point. I've only made people like you. Some are worse, many are better, but this is about the way people are. As an act of faith, will you find some other human being who is just like you with whom you can share yourself as an act of faith in Me? Do it for my sake, not for theirs."

I finally did open myself to another person for the first time at midnight in a dormitory room in a theological seminary. I can remember receiving the Holy Spirit in a whole fresh new way. Old habits and old sins for which I'd been forgiven but which I had continued to practice were gone. It was the scariest thing I had ever done in my life. And it was one of the most powerful experiences that God has led me into.

The healing community

God continues to deal with people in these small clusters of community. For years I was part of a men's group in New York City. We came once a week with a brown-bag lunch to share something of the pain and the adventure of life in Christ in mid-Manhattan. One noon a member reported that the promotion he had been expecting had gone to his boss's nephew. He described this very matter-of-factly, with no emotion. Some of the group members asked him how he felt about this turn of events. "Well, I don't feel good about it," he said, "but I am a Christian and trust in God." Such calmness did not seem normal, and for the rest of the hour various men kept probing him about his feelings and his lack of anger until finally he literally screamed out, "I'm so mad I think I'll explode." "Good," said his friends. "Now you can pray about it and we can pray for you. Before God can heal hurt you've got to get the poison out of your system." Those men had no psychological training, but they were smart enough to know that when you have been bypassed and dealt with unfairly, you've got to get your feelings out or you're going to dry up and lose the gift of wholeness. Perhaps that man was saved from a premature coronary or ulcers. Who knows? Repressed anger is a powerful negative force in life.

A pastor I know told me about a lady who came to see him about joining the church. She said her doctor had sent her. Recently she had had a facelift and when her doctor dismissed her he gave her this advice: "My dear, I have done an extraordinary job on your face, as you can see in the mirror. I have charged you a great deal of money and you were happy to pay it. But I want to give you some free advice. Find a group of people who love God and who will love you enough to help you deal with all the negative emotions inside of you. If you don't, you'll be back in my office in a very short time with your face in far worse shape than before."

I know of another small group of men who meet regularly for prayer and Bible study. One member was going to have serious back surgery and he asked the group for prayers. He had spent many painful years in traction and therapy and now as a last resort had decided on corrective surgery. They prayed for him, but afterwards one member was prompted to say, "What would it feel like if you were to stop carrying around all of the problems of your family, office, friends, and, in fact, the whole world? You walk around like someone who is overburdened by problems, your own and everybody else's. You walk like you're expecting somebody to beat you up. Why don't you try standing up straight as an act of faith in Christ?"

I was told that, there and then this man straightened up and chose a new role in life. When he saw his doctor there was no further curvature of the spine and no need for corrective surgery. Such is the medically therapeutic power of a few close friends who love you and who hold you accountable for responsible behavior.

As I write this I'm a new pastor of a West Coast church. A few nights ago I went to a dinner party in the home of one of our members. We sat around the living room at card tables in random groups of four. At our table we had some remarkable conversation. One new friend was undergoing cancer therapy and finding tremendous help in some spiritual and psychological resources. A second person was talking about stress on the job. Many of his colleagues were dying prematurely because of the pressures. We talked about what one could do to handle the stresses of life. My third dinner partner talked about a new relationship that she had found with a very close friend. Where there had been anger and resentment God had brought love and belonging. The four of us talked further about loneliness, communication, divorce.

As I returned home that evening, I realized again the miracle of community. Four Christians put together at random discovered a great treasure which was Christ in one another. There would hardly be a life problem that could not have been dealt with by that group. This is the hope of the church. May the members discover again the resources they already have. As we come together, we can uncover the wisdom and the power of God buried in His people just as He has promised. To be a whole person, choosing life, we can start by opening ourselves to a handful of others. We may even become a community.

5.

Are you living by creative risk?

I am convinced that an inordinate need for safety is actually a form of mental illness.

Several years ago I was interviewing Paul Tournier about his counseling methods. In the course of our talk, I asked, "How do you help your patients get rid of their fears?" "Oh, I don't," was his immediate answer. "That which does not frighten does not have meaning. All the best things in life have an element of fear in them."

It seemed a surprising answer at the time, but I have since come to understand more of Tournier's philosophy in this area. Actually, all of us are caught somewhere between our desire for safety and security and our need to move out to new and fearful areas. We are like badminton shuttlecocks fluttering from side to side in this emotional batting about. We are urged, "Play it safe." "Don't take chances." "Don't fail." Young people are admonished by well-meaning family and friends to choose the right school, pursue a career that will be successful, join a firm that will not fail, and belong to the right clubs. Above all, "Pick the right friends—friends that will help you and enhance your career and your prestige." Small wonder so many of us might answer no to the question "Are you living by creative risk?"

There's a lot more to health than not being sick

Risky living: some heroes

And yet our real heroes are not the people living those nice, safe, comfortable lives. When I was a small boy, I attended church every Sunday at a big Gothic Presbyterian bastion in Chicago. The preaching was powerful and the music was great. But for me, the most awesome moment in the morning service was the offertory, when twelve solemn, frock-coated ushers marched in lock-step down the main aisle to receive the brass plates for collecting the offering. These men, so serious about their business of serving the Lord in this magnificent house of worship, were the business and professional leaders of Chicago.

One of the twelve ushers was a man named Frank Loesch. He was not a very imposing-looking man, but in Chicago he was a living legend, for he was the man who had stood up to Al Capone. In the prohibition years, Capone's rule was absolute. The local and state police and even the Federal Bureau of Investigation were afraid to oppose him. But singlehandedly, Frank Loesch, as a Christian layman and without any government support, organized the Chicago Crime Commission, a group of citizens who were determined to take Mr. Capone to court and put him away. During the months that the Crime Commission met, Frank Loesch's life was in constant danger. There were threats on the lives of his family and friends. But he never wavered. Ultimately he won the case against Capone and was the instrument for removing this blight from the city of Chicago. Frank Loesch had risked his life to live out his faith.

Each Sunday at this point of the service, my father, a Chicago businessman himself, never failed to poke me and silently point to Frank Loesch with pride. Sometime I'd catch a tear in my father's eye. For my dad and for all of us this was and is what authentic living is all about. The bottom line for the Christian is to take his faith into daily life and to choose the kind of creative and risky living that will help and bless others.

Perhaps the greatest aerial troupe ever to perform in a circus were the Flying Wallendas. The patriarch, Karl, recruited and trained his own family members to perform their daring acts, for which he was the architect. They were most famous for a living pyramid formed on a high wire without a net. Imagine the drama of two men, standing on a thin wire, holding up a pole which supported ultimately about ten other people.

No circus lover will ever forget the terrible day that the pyramid fell while they were performing in a midwestern town. Two performers were killed and two were injured for life. For several days the Wallendas did not perform. Then it was announced that they would perform again and that they would climax the act with a human pyramid formed by their now diminished troupe. Of course the press was on hand to photograph and report the event. At the end of the act, old Karl Wallenda relaxed and talked to the reporters. The inevitable question was, "Mr. Wallenda, what made you go back to the act after that tragic fall a few days ago?" Seemingly surprised by the question, old Karl without a moment's hesitation said, "To be on the wire is life. All else is waiting."

Programmed for safety

You don't need to be a high-wire artist to appreciate the drama of that reply. A life of safety is no life at all, whatever your vocation. Still we are programmed from an early age to start providing for a safe and secure future. Through pension funds and retirement benefits we work toward removing all the risk from our lives by the time we are 65. Yet in the three societies sociologists have studied where people normally live to 100 and frequently up to 120, there is no special treatment for the aged. There are no retirement homes where people can spend their declining years playing shuffleboard. Scientists who have studied these three societies have found they have nothing in common in terms of climate, diet, geography or lifestyle. But in all three places the inhabitants are expected to live normal lives with no cushion of safety. They continue to work, tend fields, keep shops, and make love until they suddenly die at 100 plus. I am convinced that God never invented old age. Death is His gift, but old age is man's invention. It is a cultural blight in our lifetime.

Ashley Montague, secular philosopher living in Princeton, New Jersey, who is in his eighties, says he hopes to die young at an advanced age. "Deliver me from ever becoming adultish," says Montague. He claims that kids have all the best of it. They are risk-taking, spontaneous, and enthusiastic in their approach to life. We begin early to suppress this spontaneity, telling them to "Act your age," "Grow up," "Sit down and be quiet." Montague is waging a war against the culturally induced convention of old age, and he believes that war needs to be started almost with birth.

Most children have an inborn appetite for risk and adventure, qualities that can cause their parents or grandparents a great deal of anxiety. Most of us have at some time played out a scenario something like this: You are working on the roof, cleaning the leaves from your gutter, when you decide to come down for a drink of lemonade. You come back to find little three-year-old Herman has climbed the ladder and is precariously balancing on the edge of the roof. Immediately you yell, "Now, don't panic. I'll come and get you. Don't be frightened." Herman is not at all frightened. He thinks he was made for walking on the roof. It's the most fun thing he's ever done.

As adults, we are fortunate if we can transfer our capacity for risk and adventure into more productive avenues, to our business and vocational lives. There is excitement about being in the marketplace—buying, selling, risking financially and professionally. This is sometimes why "old Dad" stays in the family business long past retirement over and against the urging of his sons and daughters. They want him to retire and take Ma down to Florida to enjoy the benefits of the sunshine and unlimited leisure. They say, "Dad, you made your bundle. Go and enjoy the fruits of your labors. We'll run the business." But old Dad isn't buying it. The adventure of living for him means buying and selling, sometimes at a large profit, sometimes at a loss. It is the risk and uncertainty of daily life in the business world that makes life exciting. For some reason a guaranteed income among the palm trees simply doesn't interest him. He doesn't want to retire from the stimulating marketplace experience where he is pitting his wits and judgment against his peers.

Manufactured risk

I had an insight into this a few years ago during my first and only visit to Las Vegas. I was doing a three-day workshop on personal living at the Convention Center with Keith Miller. Each morning as we waited downstairs in front of our hotel for our ride to the Convention Center, we had a unique opportunity to observe all the arriving and departing guests. Now I had always envisioned Las Vegas as a town full of people in ten-gallon hats, flashy clothes, green eyeshades, and arm bands—in other words, people who looked like professional gamblers. Not so. The people who pulled up to our hotel each morning looked just like you and me, like the people we live next door to. I really began to wonder what attracted all these ordinary citizens to Las Vegas. And as I thought about it, I began to build a rationale. Let's say for fifty weeks a year many of these people are living lives of unrelieved boredom. They are committed to marriages that have ceased to be exciting. Having children was not the fulfilling experience they expected it to be. Their kids consider them back numbers and scarcely give them the time of day. The job has become routine. They could do it with one hand tied behind them and with half their attention. In short, they are living lives of dull routine.

When life is crushing you with its boredom how do you satisfy that innate appetite for risk and danger? You save up your money and go to Las Vegas or someplace like it and you play for big stakes for two weeks. Whether you win or lose, you are living by risk and the excitement and drama of those two weeks enable you to go back and face the old dull and boring routine for the next fifty weeks.

As I watched this never-ending procession of people checking into our hotel to gamble, I confess I was feeling somewhat superior about people who need to manufacture a little excitement in their lives. Just about then I felt the Lord pricking my balloon of self-righteousness: "Larson, what about you? Why is it a middle-aged, sophisticated, theological type like you is addicted to roller coasters? Whenever you get near an amusement park, you drag your poor wife in, plunk her down on a bench to watch people or read a book, and proceed to find the highest roller coaster in the park. You buy five tickets, sit in the front seat of the first car and yell your lungs out as you experience that first 90-mile-an-hour drop." The Lord had me. Why do I pay good money to be scared to death? Because it feels good. Somehow life is heightened by being scared to death some of the time.

During the seventies I was engaged in a research project during which I had the privilege of interviewing leading thinkers from all sorts of disciplines on the subject of human wholeness. I would always include this question in my interview: "What ingredients of wholeness would be common to anybody in any culture or society of the world?" The answers were invariably cautious and implied that wholeness or normalcy varied considerably from culture to culture. But if I pressed, these experts almost without exception agreed about one particular ingredient. In various forms I heard: "A healthy person is someone who can choose risk and danger."

A few years ago I had a doctor who seemed to subscribe to this theory. At a checkup just before my forty-fifth birthday, I was told that my main problem was an attack of full-blown middle-age and that I should take it very seriously. My doctor did not personally believe in middle-age, but nevertheless most people he knew fell victim to it. I asked him what he meant. "Well," he said, "middle age is a time when people are advised to take it easy. You start to live very cautiously. You avoid anything new or risky and you end up hastening the whole aging process." Then he went on to explain that when he turned forty-five he decided to reverse this process by buying an airplane and taking flying lessons. He confessed that he was a terrible pilot with no special aptitude for flying, but those two or three hours a week of danger in his life had made him a better doctor, husband, father, and Christian. He was such a poor pilot that very few of his family members or friends ever went up with him. Nevertheless, he always returned from these trips feeling alive and exhilarated.

I decided to take my doctor's advice. I couldn't afford a plane so I bought myself a motorcycle and began to commute to work on it. No matter how dull my day at the office, the ride to and from was always exciting and risky. My trip down a Maryland six-lane highway on a little Honda 175 with my briefcase strapped behind me and my necktie flying was an exhilarating and dangerous experience.

Safe or saved?

It doesn't matter where you open the Bible, you're almost sure to find an example of someone called by God to live by risk and danger. Jesus talks about this style of life in the words, "He that would save his life will lose it, but whoever loses his life for My sake will find it." Jesus calls us to lose our lives for His sake, not to become cannon fodder for God's great causes in the world. Rather, He knows that unless we begin to risk all for Him, we will lose our very lives. Putting it another way—only when we risk greatly for God can we live greatly. To conserve our lives is, in fact, to lose our lives.

To put it bluntly, being saved has nothing to do with being safe. To be saved means to be so secure in God's love, present and future, that one has no need to be safe again. Those people that we admire and honor and often envy are living lives of radical risk and danger for God's causes. I am convinced that an inordinate need for safety is actually a form of mental illness. At the same time, I acknowledge that risk for risk's sake, while it may be healthier, is not very productive. But God seems to be calling us to a life of *creative* risk. We are to be those people who are prayerfully seeking to bring about God's will and way in the affairs of men and who can give themselves to those causes with abandon.

Mother Teresa in India is a dramatic role model for this kind of living. She has chosen a life of enormous risk and danger in the worst slums of Calcutta, ministering to the hungry, the ill, and the dying. As each of us responds to our own Calcutta across the world or in our own town, we have the opportunity to serve some cause that will bless others in small and large ways, perhaps even for generations to come.

The Bible gives us very little reason to believe that being saved can be equated with being safe. In one place, we are called upon to put on the Helmet of Salvation and the Breastplate of Faith and to take up the Sword of the Spirit. Why? To do battle with the enemy, a battle in which one may very well be killed. I am always moved by Jesus' words to Peter just after his great confession, "Thou art the Christ, the Son of the Living God." Jesus said, "Thou art Peter, and upon this rock I will build my church and the gates of hell shall not prevail against it" (Matt. 16:18). Jesus gives us the image of hell as a walled fortress under siege with the people of God assaulting its walls and attacking its very doors and hell not being able to withstand our efforts. Christians, the people of God, are on the offensive against the source of evil itself, and there is no guarantee of safety in this kind of church that Jesus has promised to build.

Some years ago I lived in a New Jersey town where a new church was being built. We drove by frequently to see how the building was progressing and for a long time we couldn't figure out the plan at all. The finished product turned out to be a huge replica of Noah's Ark, which said a lot to me about the theology of that congregation. The Ark was a one-time strategy that God used to rescue a handful of His people from a worldwide flood. But to this day we find Christians with an Ark theology who huddle together in safe structures, singing hymns and listening to sermons, praying that God will protect them from the Evil World without.

We see the ultimate fruits of this kind of ark theology in the shocking story of Jonestown. In the early years of his ministry,

Jim Jones preached God's love and forgiveness in Jesus Christ. But after people responded, he led his converts to withdraw from the world and to live together in a place of safety, first in California and finally in Guyana where they could be pure and untouched by the evils around them. Well, that kind of life leads to social, spiritual and psychological cancers of all kinds. The holocaust that eventually resulted stunned the world.

The uncertain victory

We Christians have not been promised a safe and trouble-free life. Safety cannot be equated with success or deliverance. Shadrach, Meschach and Abednego *were* delivered from the fiery furnace. But their faith in God got them into that furnace in the first place. They defied the king and were to be killed. Fortunately, God had other plans and they were spared. Authentic faith does not keep us from every kind of danger or destruction. Faith does not guarantee deliverance here and now. When the early Christians of Rome defied Caesar and chose to worship Jesus, whole families of men, women and children were put into the arena with hungry lions. They prayed to their God and were *not* delivered, but their deliverance would be effected in the world to come.

The life of faith is not problem free, successful and invariably long. By faith we try to determine what God is up to with us and fling our lives with reckless abandon into the causes we think He has for us. When we do that we are in the company of the saints. Abraham and Moses never lived to see the great results God had promised them. Abraham was to have as many descendants as the grains of sand on the seashore. He died having fathered one son by Sarah. From our perspective God kept His promise because every Christian today is a spiritual descendant of Abraham as well as all of the Jews. But Abraham died unaware of his success. Moses was promised a New Land and for forty years he wandered with his people, dying before they inhabited that New Land.

There's a lot more to health than not being sick

Even our Lord Himself experienced uncertainty at the last about the ultimate success of His ministry. From the Cross He uttered the words, "My God, my God, why hast Thou forsaken Me?" He experienced the uncertain victory.

A test for decisions

Recently I saw a pamphlet entitled "The Test of Faith." I suppose the test of faith is not to worry about passing the test of faith. Of course no one ever has enough faith. But faith means not worrying about having enough faith. What about the test of faith for your life and mine? It seems to me we will have many watersheds in our lives when we are given two choices. One course is fairly safe and the other seems to be a high-risk adventure. By instinct, most of us choose the safe, secure path.

I learned to ski in middle years, thanks to our children. (They can be credited with getting us into all kinds of new areas where my wife and I would not normally be at "our time of life.") In skiing, one of the first things I learned was to lean away from the hill on the turns. It was also one of the hardest things to do; when you are a thousand feet up in the air on what seems like an almost perpendicular slope full of icy moguls, instinctively you feel safer leaning toward the hill. You have to go against your instincts and lean out over that precipitous descent if you are to survive. That's a lesson I try to remember as I come to the personal watersheds of my life. I have to fight my instinctive desire for safety and comfort if I am to get out on the risky and dangerous trails God has in mind for me.

Recently I made a radical job change. For six years I made a living as a writer and lecturer. I had almost total control of my time and my schedule. This year I accepted a call back into a very busy pastorate. I struggled with the decision for a long time. I asked advice from my children—two said don't go and one said go. I asked advice from three of my best friends—two said go, and one said don't. It was a stalemate. In the midst of this indecision I read again in Acts of the conversion of the Apostle

Paul. On the way to Damascus, Paul, formerly known as Saul of Tarsus, is blinded and made physically ill by a vision of Christ. He is taken to a house in the city where he is waiting for someone to come and deliver him.

At the same time, the Lord appears to Ananias, a sandalmaker and a believer. Ananias is praying when he hears a message that he is to go directly to Straight Street and look up someone named Paul. Ananias protests, as well he might. I can imagine him saying something like this: "Lord, have you read the newspapers? Don't you know that Saul of Tarsus is here in Damascus to kill people like me who believe in You? He is a vehement anti-Christian."

The Lord reassures Ananias, "I have prepared him. You will be the instrument for his deliverance. Go." So Ananias sets out for Straight Street. But, if he is like me, he is still questioning his guidance. At one corner he has to make the final decision: to the right, the sandal factory and a day doing his usual job; to the left, Straight Street and Saul. He may have stood at that street corner a long time hoping the Lord would speak to him one more time. Perhaps he was mistaken about hearing the Lord earlier in his room. Maybe it really wasn't the Lord at all but the results of a Kosher dill pickle he ate the night before, and in his misguided delusions, he will go to Straight Street and be killed by this anti-Christian fanatic. If Ananias does the instinctive thing that will keep him safe, he will not go. On the other hand, if the Lord does want him to go and see Paul, and in fact Paul is prepared for his visit, Ananias will be the hinge on which a great door of history will swing for all time. Even if he's mistaken about his guidance, if he goes in faith, he believes God will use even his error. If God wants him to go and he doesn't, he has missed his great opportunity. Of course, he decides to go.

Ananias's story helped me make my own decision. The easy and safe thing would be to stay where I was, doing something I was comfortable in. The new opportunity had all kinds of possibility for risk and failure. But I realized that even should the move prove a mistake for me and for those calling me, God could still use that mistake. Not to go might mean missing the great opportunity God had for me. I went and I am writing this book from that place.

It's taken me a long time to learn this lesson in my own life. If I am not certain about God's will, I need to fight against my instinctive need for safety and well-being and trust the fact that God wants to give me life. I've come to believe it would be a good idea for everyone to change jobs every seven years—or at least to change the way one does one's job. There's something magic about this seven-year cycle. In a seven-year time period every cell in your body has been replaced. As I look back over my own life, I am aware that my own job situation has changed radically just about every seven years, and I would recommend it. I especially recommend changing jobs if you're a great success in your present job. Once you've succeeded, your creative powers may become somewhat diminished.

I think it's important to see that God calls us to choose creative risk in many areas, not just in terms of career. Perhaps it's most difficult in relationships to risk saying to those closest to you things like, "I was wrong." Or "I love you." Or "I need you." Those are scary words.

Risking at any age

The ability to choose creative risk has nothing to do with age. Maggie Kuhn started the Gray Panthers because she believed that people in their seventies and eighties could become some of the most creative people in our time and a political force for good. I know many young people today who are choosing difficult and low-paying careers in areas in which they feel they can make some vital contribution. I read an article lately that reinforced the idea that it's never too late to try new ventures full of creative risks. Young people who feel inexperienced or old people who feel over the hill need not feel intimidated the article said, and it cited some encouraging statistics: Ted Williams at age forty-two slammed a home run in his last official time at bat;

Mickey Mantle, age twenty, hit twenty-three home runs his first full year in the major leagues; Golda Meier was seventy-one when she became Prime Minister of Israel; William Pitt II was twenty-four when he became Prime Minister of Great Britain. George Bernard Shaw was ninety-two when one of his plays was first produced. Mozart was just seven when his first composition was published. Benjamin Franklin was a newspaper columnist at sixteen and a framer of the Constitution when he was eighty-one. You are never too young or too old to choose to live by creative risk.

Finally let's remember that some of you reading this chapter are people who instinctively love risk and danger and choose to live this way most of the time. You don't need this chapter. But others of you really need to choose life in this area. You need to reverse one of the most deadly forces in your life—your inordinate need for safety. Ultimately, that safety is a prison. Let God help you to risk creatively, for he (she) who would lose his (her) life, will save it.

6.

Are you excited about your future?

We Christians, of all people, have a reason to hope. Hope is a gift of God based on the belief that God created us and is our friend and helper. If I believe in a God who cares about me and enters into my life, then my future is truly unlimited. If I am an accident of creation or a biological mistake, then I have no reason to think I will be anything other than what I have always been. If I am God's child, I can get my act together and begin to reverse what up to now may have been an unproductive and unpromising record.

One of the wellest and happiest people that I know is a new friend who is a very senior citizen, now almost blind and living on a very modest income. It's fun to be around this man because he is excited about his future. Chronologically, he cannot have too many years left at best. But he believes in what those years can be and what he can become in those years. My friend is a jazz buff, a saxophone player, and a songwriter. He has composed literally hundreds of songs. As I was writing this chapter, he handed me his newest, "I'll Love You Forever as I Love You Today."

I happen to like his music, but to the best of my knowledge, though he has copyrighted each song, he has never had one published or played publicly by anyone other than himself. But he keeps on writing. He continues to believe that the next song will surely be a best seller.

Hope: the vital ingredient

Well, whether it is or not, my friend is excited about his future and that's what this chapter is about. You cannot be a whole person—a well person—unless you are excited about your future. If you're not excited about your future, then you are defeated and in despair. It seems there is no middle ground. If you are excited about your future, whatever your age and circumstances, your body responds positively. If you're not excited about your future, that state of hopelessness promotes a climate in which serious physical, emotional, and spiritual problems can develop.

During a week at the famous Menninger Foundation, I asked some of the staff to identify the single most important ingredient in the treatment of the emotionally disturbed. I was told that the entire staff was unanimous in singling out *hope* as the most important factor in treatment. They went on to confess that they don't really know how to give hope to a patient. It is a spiritual and elusive gift. Nevertheless, they could discern immediately when a patient turns that crucial corner in treatment and realizes that he does not have to be what he has been before.

A simple definition of hope is this: to believe that good things are about to happen. Our hope for the future determines our course of action in the present, just as our present plays a powerful role in determining our future.

Facts or feelings

In our practical American culture we tend to trust those who deal in hard facts rather than those dreamers and visionaries who see great things for the future. Our heritage is to "stick with the facts." We are people who want to know "the bottom line." But today some of our leading scientists are encouraging a rediscovery of another kind of knowledge. Neurological researchers have found that the human brain is really twins, with a left side and a right side that are mirror images of each other. They tell us that the left side of the brain controls cognitive thinking. With the left side of the brain we add up numbers and think through problems of logic. The right side of the brain is the artistic or intuitive side. This side of the brain makes decisions on the basis of unprovable dreams and visions rather than reason.

Science is telling us that this kind of information is just as valid. We Americans have often been crippled because we have been relying so heavily on the logical left side of the brain. If we make all our life-changing decisions on the basis of logical facts, then we *are* imprisoned by our track record. As we make decisions more intuitively we begin to move into possibility thinking, the whole area of dreams and visions.

Business is now trying to train those top executives who plot and chart the course of empires to use both sides of the brain. To make decisions based on logic only is limiting.

When I was a small boy the adults around me were singing a song which invariably brought tears to their eyes. I still remember the words, "When I grow too old to dream, I'll have you to remember. . . . For when I grow too old to dream your love will live in my heart." I want to tell you that when you "grow too old to dream" you are too old! Dreams and visions are the stuff of life. Our dreams and visions make us excited about the future and therefore about the present. If you're too old to dream—you're simply too old.

A time for dreams

Paul Tournier told me years ago the secret of his life was the special "quiet time" he and his wife had each morning when they listened to God. He claimed God used that time to direct him in all sorts of areas; with his patients, his wife, the writing of his many books. He is now in his eighties and his lovely Nellie has been dead for almost six years. I saw him recently in Munich, and asked if he was still observing this custom.

My wife, Hazel, and I were having dinner with him at the time. Pushing his chair back from the table, he produced a large notebook and opened it for me. It was his quiet-time book, crammed with narrowly spaced handwriting. He told us he could not continue without that time of listening each day and that God has been giving him guidance in that morning time for almost fifty years now. He confided shyly, "I meet God and Nellie every morning to listen to God's dreams and visions for my life."

God can give us new dreams and visions at any age, and any

circumstance. Frank Laubach, founder of the Christian Literacy Crusade, is surely one of God's most unusual and effective servants in our century. At forty-five, Frank Laubach was a theological seminary professor and a missionary in the Philippines. He was next in line for the presidency at that seminary, but when the incumbent president retired, the seminary board chose somebody else. Laubach took off for the hills to sulk, just like some of the Biblical characters before him. He was mad about the unfairness of life and the injustices of God. At midlife, he was a failure by his own standards.

But while he was there God spoke to him, "Frank, you can change. I have great things for you to do." Subsequently, God gave Laubach the creative key to teaching hundreds of millions of people throughout the world to read for the first time. He is the father of the modern literacy movement and one of the most pivotal people in our time. As a Christian missionary he agreed to help non-Christian governments set up literacy programs for which he could supply the materials—and, of course, he supplied portions of the Bible. This man opened up the pages of the Bible to literally hundreds of millions of people. He refused to be a victim of his past failures. He had hope for what God could do through him in the second half of his life.

The power of hope

One of my all-time favorite musical plays is *Man of La Mancha*. I cannot see the play nor hear the music from it without being moved. The story's hero is a crazy old man suffering from what we would now call senile psychosis. The action takes place a hundred years past the age of chivalry and there are no knights anymore. But, thinking he is one, Don Quixote puts on a strange suit of armor and rides forth into the world to battle evil and protect the weak and powerless. He brings along his funny little servant Sancho Panza as his squire. When they arrive at a broken down old inn used by mule traders, Don Quixote calls the innkeeper the lord of a great castle. The innkeeper tells him he is bonkers. In the inn he meets the most miserable human being imaginable, a pathetic orphan girl who does the most menial chores and is used sexually by every mule trader passing through. He pronounces this wretched girl the great lady, Dulcinea, and he begs for her handkerchief as a token to take into battle. She reacts with fury.

At the end of the play the old man about to die is no longer suffering from these delusions. In a moving scene, all the people he has renamed appear at his bedside and beg him not to change. His excitement about their future has transformed them and they have become the people that this insane visionary saw in them. This story moves us because we recognize the truth of the message. Our dreams and our hopes are powerful motivating forces in the lives of those around us.

One of the basic ideas we learn from the Bible is that life is not always fair or logical. We live in a spiritual world that defies hard facts and logical conclusions. In this life, good is not always rewarded nor evil always punished. The Bible often presents us with mysteries that are far from logical.

In Ecclesiastes 9:11 God says to us, "The race is not to the swift, nor the battle to the strong, nor bread to the wise, nor riches to men of understanding, nor favor to men of skill; but time and chance happen to them all" (RSV). We live in an unpredictable world where anything can happen. By human effort, we cannot understand why things are as they are nor can we foresee what will yet be. As we live in hope, we can tap into spiritual forces that can reverse our own destiny and the destiny of those around us. If we're really in touch with God, we're excited about the future. And I believe we can only be whole and well persons if we have hope for our futures, if we really believe "it's never too late."

An unlimited future

Even business people are moving away from the kind of decision-making based solely on hard facts. They're saying instead, "If you can imagine it, you can possess it; if you can dream it, you can become it. If you can envision it, you can attain it. If you can picture it, you can achieve it." This kind of unstructured thinking is desperately needed today in the scientific world. I have been told that although we now have almost unlimited capabilities to produce whatever we can envision, we lack scientists with an excitement about the future who can provide those visions.

How indebted we are in this area to someone like Jules Verne, the novelist of fifty years ago. With prophetic insight, he wrote about submarines that traveled under the polar icecap at sea and spaceships that flew to the moon and beyond. His excitement about the future fueled the creative capacities of scientists who eventually built the incredible wonders he envisioned. In our generation, there has been by contrast a procession of gloomy, prophet-type novelists who believe we are locked into a predictable future based on both our past and our current direction. George Orwell's *1984* of thirty years ago and *The Greening of America* a decade ago are two pointed examples.

Futurologists are presently apologizing for having given us mistaken information. They had been making projections about what life will be like on this planet based on past performance. They'd been charting things like birth rates, death rates, food production, oil consumption, divorce rates and disease potential, all of which had been based on the statistics and growth rates of the past. Our politicians have tried to make provision for the future on the basis of their information.

Now the futurologists tell us that they *cannot* predict the future. They had assumed that the future was linear, when actually it is systemic. Linear is the adjective describing action that follows the curve of a graph, progressing along a line, whereas, systemic refers to the presence of multiple options at any given point in time. We have multiple options, and that means our future is systemic. The future will be what we want to make of it. Corporately the future of the world depends on whether we are excited about the years ahead or stoically resigned to more of the same.

Hope gets results

The contagious power of hope has been tested in the classrooms of the state of California. Some years ago, all of the students of a random number of classes were given some tests by state psychologists. They were actually "Mickey Mouse" tests, proving nothing. Half a dozen students were then arbitrarily picked from each of the classes, and their teachers were told something like this: "Our tests indicate that these are the students who have great potential this year. They're ready to blossom academically. Keep a special eye on them to see if our tests are accurate."

You can believe that those students were given very special attention that year. The records prove that, almost without exception, those students did unusually well simply because their teachers had an inordinate amount of hope for their success. When you expect great things for yourself or others, you are setting forces in motion that work toward producing those great things.

We Christians, of all people, have a reason to hope. Hope is a gift of God based on the belief that God created us and is our friend and helper. If I believe in a God who cares about me and enters into my life, then my future is truly unlimited. If I am an accident of creation or a biological mistake, then I have no reason to think I will be anything other than what I have always been. If I am God's child, I can get my act together and begin to reverse what up to now may have been an unproductive and unpromising record.

In Proverbs, we are told, "Where there is no vision, the people perish" (KJV). And God is the giver of those visions. When we lose sight of God's vision for us personally and corporately, we are defeated before we begin. The Old Testament gives us many examples of this truth operating in the lives of the early Israelites. Battles were won or lost on the basis of their vision or lack of it. They were repeatedly warned against trafficking in horses and chariots—the ancient counterpart of missiles, submarines, and long-range bombers. Hope is the essential theme of the Bible. God-given hope changes the fate of nations and transforms individuals. Today's English version of the Bible translates Romans 8:24 in this way: "For it was by hope that we were saved. . . . For who hopes for something he sees? But if we hope for what we do not see, we wait for it with patience." In Corinthians 13:13 the Apostle Paul says, "So faith, hope, love abide, these three . . ." (RSV). He lists hope as one of the three greatest marks of being God's faithful people.

In touch with God's hopes

How much we need to receive God's gift of hope for our own lives. The absence of hope makes us depressed, anxious, victims of emotional stress and therefore vulnerable to mental and physical problems. In the Old Testament God spoke to the Israelites only through certain individuals. The Prophets, the Kings and the Judges passed on their visions of God to the rest of the nation. But God promised to make a new covenant with his people: "And it shall come to pass afterward," God declared, "that I will pour out my spirit upon all flesh; and your sons and your daughters shall prophesy, your old men shall dream dreams, your young men shall see visions: and also upon the servants and upon the handmaids in those days will I pour out my spirit" (KJV). Jesus came to fulfill that prophecy. Through His life, death, and presence now through the Holy Spirit, all of us have access to the dreams and visions God has for us. God has promised that His Spirit will give us dreams and visions for our own lives as well as for His church, our society, and the world. Our hope is not based upon facts. It is based on God Himself.

All of the great heroes of the Bible were people in touch with God's vision for their lives. Because of hope, Abraham left all the comfort and security of his home and set out to establish a new nation. Through hope, Abraham endured all the hardships of his pilgrimage that are recorded in the book of Genesis. God gave Moses a vision at the burning bush. God gave him hope for what could be done through him for the people of Israel. For forty years, Moses was faithful to that vision through horrendous adversities and in spite of being misunderstood by his followers. The Prophets are in the same tradition. Though they are a diverse group in terms of message and style, all were full of hope that God would bless and deliver Israel.

An exile with hope

My favorite hoper in the Bible is the Apostle John. The youngest of Jesus' disciples, he outlived the others. As an old man, he was still so full of hope in Jesus and so radical in his obedience to Him, that he became politically troublesome. Civil authorities exiled him to the most remote place they could think of—the island of Patmos in the Aegean Sea. Patmos is both beautiful and bleak, its hillsides partly covered with scrub growth and partly barren. The entire island is one steep hill, and two-thirds of the way up is the cave where John lived out his last years. It is now a Greek Orthodox shrine, tended by a handful of faithful monks. Through the mouth of the cave you can see across the little island to the Aegean Sea. It is moving to imagine John living there through his last years, cut off from everything he knew or loved, every vestige of civilization as it was known then. Yet from that remote place, John saw everything: "Then I saw a new heaven and a new earth; for the first heaven and the first earth had passed away, and the sea was no more. And I saw the holy city, new Jerusalem, coming down out of heaven from God, prepared as a bride adorned for her husband; and I heard a great voice from the throne saying, 'Behold, the dwelling of God is with men. He will dwell with them, and they shall be his people, and God himself will be with them; he will wipe away every tear from their eyes, and death shall be no more, neither shall there be mourning or crying or pain any more, for the former things have passed away'" (Rev. 21:1–4, RSV).

Having no personal future in this life, John was nevertheless excited about the future. God gave him the gift of hope. Being nowhere, he saw everything. Without hope we can stand in the middle of one of the great capitals of the world and see nothing. All we see is pollution, crime, unemployment, and man's inhumanity to man. With God we can be in the most remote place in the world in the middle of a seemingly hopeless exile and we can have hope about what God is doing in our lives and in the world.

New hope for ourselves

I have hope that God is going to be able to do something new in your life and mine no matter where we are—or who we are. Many of us are in despair because we don't like who we are. The person inside is quite different from the person the world sees. Communication is often difficult because the real me is not the person you see and relate to. My outward personality has become a cloak or coat that keeps you from really seeing me. I may feel you like me because of my personality, and I'm fearful that the real me may offend you.

Let's put it this way. When we were small children we tried on different personality coats. We tried lots of methods of getting our needs met. We may have been alternately loud and demanding, shy or withdrawn. We may have tried being cute for awhile. At other times we were belligerent show-offs or know-it-alls, intellectuals or slick operators who know how to manipulate parents and teachers. As we were experimenting with these different coats, one day the tragically unexpected happened. The zipper got stuck and we couldn't get the darn thing off. Suddenly we were stuck in the last coat we tried on, and we are still wearing it at nineteen or thirty-five or fifty-two. We are stuck with being the withholder, the sulker, the critical person, the pleaser, the know-it-all, the wise guy or the cynic. The coat has not fit us for years but we don't know how to get it off.

When God intervenes in your life and mine he says, "Let me help you take that coat off." I can't believe my good fortune. Is God really offering me a chance to get the coat off? I remind Him that the zipper is stuck. He says, "I'll unzip it." And that's exactly what He does. Like Zacchaeus or the woman by the well in Samaria or the wise theologian Nicodemus, I am now in the presence of God and I find I can work the zipper and take that personality off. At that point God says, "I've got a whole bunch of coats. See if you can find one that fits you better—one that we will both like." I can try to find one that expresses who I really am inside and I am free to wear that coat as long as it fits. But I can even trade that one in when it no longer reflects who I am.

God can bring about this kind of integration. My outside personality will reflect the real person. I am no longer many personalities like the Gadarene demoniac. I can wear my new coat with integrity and joy in every situation. If you like the me you now see, you are really my friend. If you don't, I am free to move on and find those who will accept and love me as I am.

New hope for our circumstances

But let's say that even after God has come into your life and integrated it, and you are more at home with who you are, you may still have a hard time feeling excited about your future. Perhaps you're overwhelmed by your past record; you have simply blown it too many times. You have a history of addictions or dissipation or irresolution or procrastination—the list goes on and on. If that's the case, read again the story of King David. Few people had a worse track record. But God called him a man after His own heart.

Perhaps you are hopeless about the future because there are people in your life who are "out to get you." They won't cheer if you succeed and they'll rejoice if you fail. The truth is that when you and I begin to follow God's guidance for our lives, He can use even our enemies to accomplish His will for us. Joseph was sold into slavery by his brothers, who were jealous of him, and with good reason. Years later, he has become the governor in Egypt and has saved the Egyptians from seven years of famine by storing up grain during the seven good years. His brothers, who had committed this crime against him, come to Egypt to ask help from Pharaoh and his storehouses of grain. When they discover that their fate is in Joseph's hands, they think they are done for. He will surely deny them food, perhaps even kill them. Instead, Joseph says poignantly, "You meant it for evil, but God meant it for good." He never denies the evil that was in their hearts. They still have to answer to God for that. But Joseph believed that God could use even his enemies to accomplish His purposes.

Reading this, you may be thinking you have no enemies. If so, I believe you are in sad shape. We have a word for those people who think everyone is against them: paranoia. But there is no word for those who think that everybody loves them, and that is a sickness just as real. Everyone does not love us. We cannot live without raising the enmity of some—especially if we care passionately about certain causes or issues. But we can still be excited about our futures because even our enemies can be God's instruments for constructive change in all sorts of situations.

The right credentials

Finally, we limit our future when we hesitate to do what God has called us to do because we feel inadequate, because we do not have the training, the credentials, the experience. Our patron saint could be Amos, the prophet. Amos came down from the rural areas to the great city of Jerusalem to challenge the king. He flatly told the king that he was out of sync with God's direct will. Before he gave the king this message from the Lord he stated his credentials: "I am no prophet nor the son of a prophet. I am simply Amos, a fig picker from Tekoa." When God gives you a mandate, believe that He is able to accomplish through you those things that need to be done and that He will give you the wisdom you need for the job.

I used to live near Fort Myers, Florida, which was the winter home of Thomas Edison for almost fifty years. Edison has been credited with inventing the twentieth century. In terms of practicality, certainly his greatest invention was the light bulb. But Edison takes no credit for making the light bulb available to the world. He simply invented the first one. It did not last very long or give enough light and it was too expensive. A man named Thomas Coolidge spent seven years working on the light bulb trying to find a filament that would make it more useful and practical. At that time, tungsten was the only element that could work as a filament, but scientists declared it was not sufficiently malleable and therefore could not be used. When Coolidge finally succeeded in his efforts, he was questioned about how he was able to make tungsten work. He said, "It was because I was not a metallurgist. Had I been a metallurgist, I would have known that the task was impossible."

On his twentieth birthday, our youngest son bought himself his first ten-speed bicycle with a tax refund from the Internal Revenue Service. The day after he bought his new bike, an all-Florida professional bike race was held in our town. Mark, along with two friends, decided to enter. I tried to discourage him. I told him bike racing was very sophisticated and he was foolish to try it with no training. "But it will be a good experience," he said.

He returned that night with the first-place cup. Needless to say, we were astounded. I asked him what happened. "Well," he said, "I know long distance bike racing is very tricky. You have to learn to pace yourself carefully and make your move at the right time. Since I didn't know exactly what to do, I just started out pedaling as fast as I could—and nobody ever passed me."

The moral is obvious. No one is too inexperienced. No one is too young or too old. We can all have an exciting future. When we cease to be excited about our futures we have lost touch with God. Find Him again, and hope will spring in our hearts. We can tap into the dreams and visions He has for us.

7.

Do people feel important around you?

Life breaks down not so much because of the terrible things that happen to us. Life breaks down because so few good things have happened to us. None of us has enough good things happen to us. Just a few along the way can be like branches we can cling to as we climb up a mountain trail. No matter how steep the ascent, we can make it, if from time to time along the trail someone communicates to us that he or she loves us and therefore we are important.

"Love or perish!" Do you remember who said that? It wasn't Jesus and it wasn't some preacher. It was a clinical psychologist named Smiley Blanton who wrote a book by that title some years ago. He says those are our only options and I happen to believe him. Karl Menninger, one of our most honored psychiatrists, said years ago, "Love is the medicine for the sickness of the world." At the root of most of our problems, he would say, is the inability to give or receive love. The problem is, what does one do to become a lover? What does love look like? What does love feel like? How do I know if I am a lover? In other words, what is the clinical shape of love? If I am to communicate my love to another person in negotiable terms, what kind of behavior is required?

One simple test is the question posed in our chapter title. Let's say that right now you're sitting across from Doctor V., whose interview with his patient Paul we described in chapter 1. He has asked, "Do people feel important around you?" Your answer will tell you whether or not you are communicating love. You can't convince me you're a lover if the people you're trying to love do not feel important around you. If you're on the receiving end of my love in any kind of relationship—family, friend, or lover— you ought to feel important around me. That's what love is all about.

Love—a scarce commodity

This fall I was asked to speak to the faculty of church school teachers in my new parish about effective Christian education. As a learning exercise, I asked those seventy teachers to think about the most effective teacher they had ever had. What teacher had been most used by God to help them discover their potential and become the persons they were now? Next, I asked them to describe the behavior of that unusual teacher. Then we shared a composite list of all the results, a list describing the qualities of those great teachers in our lives. Here's what we found out: great teachers listen a lot; they trust their students; they spend time with them; they share their own problems; they visit the students in places other than the classroom; they point out skills and talents of which the students themselves are unaware.

Actually, the list was much longer than that. Every one of the behaviors, remembered in some cases for almost forty years, were behaviors designed to make the student feel important. Apparently this is what great teaching is all about, and, in fact, great teaching is really love in action. Arthur Combs, head of the School of Education at the University of Florida in Gainesville, told a group of educators some years ago that there are two requirements for good teachers. They must love themselves and love their students. If those two qualities are present learning is inevitable. A good college can give additional skills to that kind of a teacher, but without those two qualities, the skills will be of little effect.

Tragically, most of us have been exposed to very few parents or teachers or friends who have the capacity or the will to make us feel important. Even one or two such people in your life can make an enormous difference. Psychiatrists' offices are full of people who have been emotionally crippled because they have never been loved in this way.

In a small group some years ago, we were all talking about our growing-up years. The question was asked, "When was the first time you knew you were important and had worth?" Several of us answered the question before my friend Walter had his turn. "You know, I was raised in a fine Christian family," he said. "There were six boys and my parents were wonderful people. They took us to church several times on Sunday and often during the week. We had a family altar and we prayed every day. The Bible was the center of our life. But, you know, I was twelve years old before I realized that my father knew my name. He was a hard man to please. We all did chores around the house and they were never done to please him. Most of his conversation consisted of, 'You didn't cut the lawn right!' or 'You left the basement door open,' or 'You forgot to cut the wood.' I thought I was just one of his six sons, but when I was 12 years old he suddenly called me by name in the middle of a weeding project. 'Walter,' he said, 'You've left a lot of those weeds.' I was so thrilled that he knew my name. I thought I was just No. 3. Suddenly I had worth as a person."

Apparently, for that parent, love did not require getting intimately involved with his children. I'd call it parenting with sort of a Playboy philosophy. That philosophy suggests that sex is something you do with an object. For heaven's sake, don't get emotionally involved with another person. That's what your parents and grandparents did, and look where it got them—families and babies. Sex is a simple normal act just like brushing your teeth or going to the bathroom. Find somebody that turns you on and have sex. Go through life using people as objects. This self-indulgent philosophy is all part of the same tragic lie that leaves people so crippled. We need to know that we are loved. If we are loved we will feel important. And that's the message that God's been trying to communicate since He invented the first people back in the Garden of Eden.

A capacity for miracles

The power of love is an important part of our folk wisdom. We read fairy stories about princesses in suspended animation who can only be awakened by love's first kiss. Little children run

107

to an adult they love with a hurt finger or a cut knee crying, "Kiss it and make it well." They know instinctively that love is therapeutic.

Jesus said, "These things that I do shall ye do also, and greater things, because I go to my Father" (John 14:12). It is recorded that He performed many miracles. He healed the sick, opened the eyes of the blind and raised the dead. What greater things than these are there? Perhaps one of these "greater things" is our potential for transforming others by the power of our love. One of my all-time heroines performed this sort of a miracle. She is the teacher, Annie Sullivan, who took on the multiply handicapped child, Helen Keller. This little girl seemed hopelessly locked inside herself. Unable to talk, see, or hear, she had become a hostile, untamed, rebellious animal. With tough love, Annie Sullivan fought her way into Helen's life and released from the prison of her self one of the most beautiful and gifted women of all time. I think this is an example of the "greater things" Jesus prophesied. You and I have the capacity for miracles of this kind if we learn how to be lovers and begin to communicate to others that they are important to us and of supreme worth in the eyes of God.

Earlier in this chapter I quoted Karl Menninger's statement that "love is the medicine for the sickness of the world." The medical establishment as a whole is beginning to believe that as well and is increasingly acknowledging the power of love to heal the body and the mind. Some of the first startling statistics on this phenomenon came years ago from a study done in a foundling home in Brazil. The records indicate that the infants there received excellent care. The conditions were sanitary. There was an adequate staff to provide all physical and dietary needs. But there was not enough staff to provide physical love, to simply hold the babies, touch them, and play with them. Most of the babies died before the end of the first year. "Love or perish!" is more than a dramatic phrase. It is a scientific truth. Love is an essential ingredient of life, and those who are denied love, assuming that they survive at all, usually end up handicapped and damaged in some way.

A poignant drama

Our feelings of no worth can begin very early. About a year ago I was giving a four-day lectureship in a midwestern town. My wife and I stayed in a lovely hotel not far from the sponsoring church. Between the morning and evening lecture, we had the afternoons free. Since it was early spring and the weather was delightful, we spent those afternoons sitting by our hotel pool. I would work on my evening talk while Hazel read. We usually had the place to ourselves, but one afternoon we found another family there. A little girl about five was playing in the pool while her family sat nearby—obviously her mother, grandmother, and grandfather. I deduced that the mother and daughter had come for a visit with the grandparents.

For about half an hour this little girl dove and splashed and swam, yelling all the while, "Granddaddy, granddaddy, look at me. See what I can do! Look what I have learned! Granddaddy, watch this!" Unfortunately, granddaddy was so busy talking to his daughter and his wife he never once looked her way. Clearly the little girl was playing her life to granddaddy; he was her most important audience. Unable to watch this scene any longer, I put my notebook down and went over to the little girl. I said, "How about showing me what you can do?" She looked up with some annoyance. "Oh, well, all right—" She took a quick dive into the pool and swam across. But as she climbed out again, she resumed her pleas, "Granddaddy! Granddaddy! Come see what I can do!"

She didn't want my attention; she wanted granddaddy's. I would be willing to bet that granddaddy would have given his life for that little girl. I'm sure she was the apple of his eye. Perhaps he was hard of hearing or simply absorbed in the delight of visiting with his daughter; I don't know the circumstances. I only

109

know that too many experiences like that will destroy a little girl's sense of worth. If enough people ignore her needs to feel loved and important she might very well end up, at thirty or forty, in some psychiatrist's office talking about her problems.

Life breaks down not so much because of the *terrible* things that happen to us. Life breaks down because *so few good* things have happened to us. None of us has enough good things happen to us. Just a few along the way can be like branches we can cling to as we climb up a mountain trail. No matter how steep the ascent, we can make it, if from time to time along the trail someone communicates to us that he or she loves us and therefore we are important.

Effective helpers

That's the message a good therapist can give us. Modern psychotherapy tells us that a good counseling relationship is the result of what is called the therapeutic triad. An effective counselor—psychiatric, psychological, or pastoral; directive or nondirective; Christian or secular—has three qualities, all more important than personality theories and counseling methods. And what are they? The first is empathy—the ability to feel whatever it is the counselee is feeling. The second is personal honesty. An effective counselor is honest about his or her feelings and in touch with them while the counseling process is going on. The third quality is the one we're talking about in this chapter—love. The scientific world is a bit leery of that term. They call it "nonpossessive warmth." That's exactly the kind of love we're talking about. Love is not manipulating somebody to get him or her around to your point of view. God loves us with no strings, and I'm sure this is the way he wants us to love others. It's the kind of love that makes you and me feel mighty important, no matter how dumb our behavior may have been up to now.

If, as we're told, professional therapists who have these qualities become the most effective helpers, then the implication is that even people without scientific training who have these three qualities can be in a therapeutic relationship with others and be effective and enabling counselors.

Loving and liking

In one sense, "love or perish" is at the very heart of what God has been trying to say to man throughout the Bible and for centuries since. Jesus says, "By this shall all men know that you are my disciples if you love one another" (John 13:35). His great commandment to us is to "love one another as I have loved you" (John 15:12). In 1 John 4:20 we read, "How can you say that you love God, whom you have not seen, if you don't love your brother whom you have seen?" The Bible also tells us to love our enemies. Why? Not for our enemy's sake but for our own sakes. Our resentments and hatreds set forces in motion that undermine our physical health and our psychological well-being. You may think it is impossible to love your enemy. It's important here to understand the difference between loving and liking. You and I have no control over whom we like. Liking is some kind of magnetism or personality meshing that is mysterious and beyond our control. I can't choose whom I will like. Certain people turn me on, and I never seem to get enough of them. Other people turn me off very quickly, and I am happy to leave them. I don't believe God wants us to feel guilty about those we don't like; rather, we are to be grateful for those whom we do like. But liking has nothing to do with love and we can love anyone. We can love those we do not like, because love is simply acting in somebody else's best interest. I can honor those persons whom I do not happen to like by letting them know that I care about them.

I have a friend who is a gifted pastor. He has a great capacity for honoring the people who disagree with him theologically, politically, or socially. He is courageous about his beliefs and willing to disagree publicly with those who oppose him. But he never minimizes the people with whom he's in sharp disagreement. They are still his friends. He plays golf with them, has lunch with them. In short, he honors them and makes them feel important. He never conceals the fact that he does not agree with them.

We have said that we can't like everyone but we can love everyone, even those who are withholding love from us and who seem to be obstacles to our advancement. As Christians, I believe the most important thing is for each of us to *want* to be a lover. Jesus Himself has promised to make me a lover. If there is somebody whom I consciously do not love, I can ask for a heart transplant that will let God do the thing in me that I cannot do for myself. I can ask God to motivate me to begin to act in a positive and helpful way toward this person whom I do not happen to like.

A strategy for loving

But that's just the first step. You and I have known people who have had this kind of transformation in their hearts and they suddenly have new love for those people with whom they've been having a difficult time—be it child, wife, husband, friend, or business associate. But their strategy for expressing this new love is all wrong. They continue to behave in ways that turn the other person off. Their love is not expressed in terms that are meaningful to the other person. Jesus modeled a strategy for loving that helps the other person feel important. That is the bottom line of love. As you read the Gospels, you realize how much time Jesus spent with individuals and how greatly affirmed were those people with whom He spent time. Some were healed, some were enlightened. Some were challenged and some were reconciled. But all felt important around Him—the outcast woman by a well in Samaria, the rich young ruler, the theologian who came by night, the crazy man from the hills of Gadara, the little group of fishermen and tax collectors who traveled with Him.

Let us look at the shape of love as He models it. First of all,

Jesus listened to people. Read the Gospels and see how He continually asks questions of people and listens to their answers. He wants to know what they are thinking about themselves or their problems or about Him and about life. If we want to make people feel important because they're important to God, there's no better way than by listening. Psychologists tell us we cannot clinically distinguish intense listening from love. It looks like the same thing whether it is or not.

It seems that many of us are so intent on telling people about ourselves and our own agenda that we have no time to listen. A couple of years ago I almost drowned in the Gulf of Mexico. I got into that predicament through a bizarre set of circumstances that I have detailed in an earlier book. Briefly, I was rescued by a tugboat crew after many harrowing hours of trying to keep afloat in wild and stormy seas. A couple of days later I met an old friend I hadn't seen in years. After we chatted a bit he said to me, "What's new with you?" I said, "Well, you won't believe this, but two days ago I almost drowned in the Gulf of Mexico. I was rescued by a tugboat after four hours in the sea."

My friend and I stood there for awhile and he didn't say anything. He was looking at his shoes. Eventually, though, he looked up and said, "By the way, how's fishing these days?" You can guess what my reaction was. To say the least I felt unloved and put down. But then I thought about the many times I had met friends and asked how they were and much later remembered words like, "My wife is sick," or, "I lost my job last week," or, "I have an operation coming up." Unfortunately, I had already dropped some pleasantry and hurried on. If I want to be a lover like Jesus—and I can be with His help—I've got to begin to listen to people and take them seriously.

Giving ourselves

Jesus models another important aspect of the shape of love. He gave himself to people. He gave His time. As busy as He must have been during those three intense years of His ministry,

113

He was interruptible. Nobody had a more pressure-packed schedule than He. As He was sought out by day or by night for quiet conversations or for healing, He gave His attention and any other agenda was postponed.

How interruptible am I? This is a really pertinent question just now. I am a busy pastor of a very active church. I have enough items on my schedule, any day, to fill up all my time. But it is possible that the most important thing God has for me on any given day is not even on my agenda. It may be the teenager who knocks at my door or a chance meeting with one of our custodial staff in the hall or a chat with some senior citizen on the way to a church meeting. Am I interruptible? Do I have time for the non-programmed things in my life? My response to those interruptions is the real test of my love. If I make the other person feel that he or she is interrupting me, then that person certainly doesn't feel important. If I can communicate that I have time for him or her—even when I don't—then I am acting in love and God may even use that response to produce the real thing.

As Christians most of us are focused on rescuing others, on helping and giving to them. Well, Jesus certainly gave of himself all the time. But as I read the record of His life on this earth, I'm aware that He was able to receive as well. He asked the Samaritan woman for water, He asked Zacchaeus for a meal for Himself and His disciples. At Gethsemane, He asked for companionship. He asked for a mule on which to ride into Jerusalem. In a relationship of love, the other person cannot feel important if I am always the giver. That person needs to give as well, and we make this possible as we ask for advice or for help with a specific task on a committee. This is the very stuff of love. A Christian is not always going about doing good. Part of the time a Christian is giving other people the chance to do good, and thereby to feel loved and of worth.

An old friend of mine, a thoracic surgeon, had a remarkable conversion in his middle life and in recent years has been trying to communicate his faith to his patients. He used to offer to pray for his patients. But now he asks them to pray for him. As he talks to them in his office, at the hospital or even on the telephone, he always ends the conversation by saying, "Will you pray for me?"

Bill confided his reason to me, "You see, I already am a very important person in the lives of my patients. They are sick and they come to me for help. If I'm going to pray for them as well as treat them medically, it really is a one-way relationship. But, Bruce, you know what a needy person I am. I need all the prayers I can get just to survive day by day. So I decided to ask my patients to do something for me, and I'm grateful if they do." How do the patients respond? Bill said, "Well, some say, 'Oh, sure, doc.' Others say, 'Yeah, I will, but will you pray for me too?' Then I say, 'You bet. I'll be glad to. I'll do it right now if you'd like.'"

Being real people

Jesus brought reality to every encounter, and that is another important dimension of love. A genuine lover is not plastic or falsely pious or always in control. Real people can get angry from time to time. Jesus got angry when He saw what was happening in God's house, and He made a whip and drove the money changers out of the Temple. My friend Charlie Shedd, Presbyterian clergyman and noted author and lecturer, tells a story I love. One morning he came down to breakfast after having had a terrible fight with his wife, Martha, the night before. For the first time in their married life, Martha was not there making breakfast. She had left the house. He found a note propped up by the sugar bowl. It said, "Dear Charlie: I hate you. (Signed) Love, Martha." That's what love is all about. Love is being able to say, "I love you." But it is also being able to say on occasion, "I hate you." If we can't express anger, we probably can't love.

We all know of rejected children whose parents have ignored or abused them. But there is another kind of rejected child—the child whose parents are too nice, too lenient, too kind and too permissive. This child is treated in a special way without the give-and-take he or she observes taking place with siblings. That specialness is perceived by the child as rejection. The parents feel puzzled since they are always so kind. But the child instinctively knows that if we are really loved by a real person there will be times of conflict and even anger.

Love requires emotion. People who are not able to express their emotions are questionable lovers. Remember that "Jesus wept" when He came to the house where his friend Lazarus had died. He loved Lazarus and his two sisters, Mary and Martha. When He came to that house of grief He joined with the rest of the household in their expression of grief.

A friend of mine, an orphan who was raised in a supposedly Christian orphanage, tells harrowing tales about his years in that inhuman and unloving home. His life was scarred by those years, but fortunately, he was adopted while still a young lad and his adoptive father became one of the great people in his life. A simple and poor man, he took this boy into his home, gave him his name, and somehow managed to reverse the damage that had been done to him. My friend is now teaching at a theological seminary and pastoring a great church. I'll always be grateful to that adoptive father who believed in him and let him know that he was of worth.

Some years back my friend, now married and the father of two children, wrote a letter to his adoptive father expressing his love and gratitude in great detail. The letter was never answered or mentioned in subsequent visits. At his adoptive father's funeral, my friend asked his mother, "Did Dad ever get my letter?" She answered, "Oh, son, you will never know what that letter meant to him. It was the greatest treasure of his life. No one ever came here to visit—friend or even bill collector—that your dad did not produce that letter and read it."

Our friend couldn't help feeling somehow cheated. His father, afraid of his own emotions, was unable ever to respond to that special letter. Had the old man been able to let his emotions out and share his feelings with his son, he would have given him a great gift.

Seeing the invisible

Perhaps most of all, Jesus had the unique quality of seeing the invisible in other people. And that is such an essential dimension of love. It's so easy for us to miss the promise of leadership in young persons. We dismiss them or don't take time with them because they are still so unformed. We ignore the aged. They can no longer be of use to us in our striving for success and status. Jesus took time for children. He took no one for granted—not the blind, the sick, the rich, or the learned. He saw the potential for wholeness and transformation in each person.

I heard about an old woman who had died in a nursing home in Scotland some years ago. She had left nothing of value, but in going through her very few possessions the nurses found a poem she had written. Here is part of it.

What do you see, nurses, what do you see?
What are you thinking when you're looking at me?
A crabby old woman not very wise,
Uncertain of habit with faraway eyes.
I'm a small child of ten with a mother and father,
Brothers and sisters who love one another,
A bride in her twenties—my heart gives a leap,
Remembering the vow that I promised to keep.
A woman of thirty, my young now grow fast,
Bound to each other with ties that should last.
At forty, my sons have grown and have gone,
But my man is beside me, to see I don't mourn.
At fifty, once more babies play around my knees;
Again we know children, my husband and me.
I'm an old woman now and nature is cruel;
'Tis her jest to make old age look like a fool.
The body it crumbles, grace and vigor depart;
There is now a stone where I once had a heart.
But inside this old carcass a young girl still dwells,
And now and again my battered heart swells.
I remember the joys, and I remember the pains;

There's a lot more to health than not being sick

> And I'm loving and living life over again.
> I think of the years all too few—gone too fast,
> And accept the stark fact that nothing can last.
> So open your eyes, nurses, open and see
> Not a crabbed old woman; look closer—see me.

That's exactly what Jesus did. He saw you and He saw me, not as we appear to others, but as we really were and are. Old or young, He saw the treasure in us and called it forth. And God calls us to be those who can see in others the true and the real and the hidden. Life has no greater adventure then to be in partnership with God in loving the world—in making the people around us feel that they are important.

8.

Do you have the courage to be happy?

Doctors have been telling me for years that "you can't kill a happy man." When I press for an explanation, they suggest that unhappiness often precedes an illness. Happy people rarely get sick and tend to recover quickly when they do get sick. The unhappy person is the target for any and every kind of illness.

What is your reaction to the question: Do you have the courage to be happy? It may seem like a foolish question since it suggests that happiness is a matter of conscious choice. Who would not choose to be happy? But, odd as it may seem, I'm convinced that there are a good many people who choose not to be happy.

It has taken me a long time to understand this mystery. I'm reminded of two women elders in a church I served many years ago. Both of these women were devout believers—generous, kind, and living seemingly blameless lives. One seemed to be a wellspring of joy and happiness. She bubbled with enthusiasm and wonder at the goodness of life. She enjoyed being alive and who she was. The second woman could be characterized best by the word *long-suffering*. She gave the impression that life was a burden and her days were full of dutiful service to be endured.

I was especially intrigued by the contrast these two elders represented. The one full of joy was a person of very modest circumstances with a sickly husband and no children. The long-suffering woman was a person of some means with a devoted husband and family, all of whom seemed to be dancing around trying to do her bidding. Happiness or the lack of it for these two women seemed to have nothing to do with the actual circumstances of their lives.

121

It seems to me our capacity for happiness is tied up inextricably with our health and well-being. Our ability to accept happiness, or actually the courage to accept it, determines greatly how well we are physically and emotionally. The ecclesiastical wisemen who drew up the Westminster Confession of Faith centuries ago had this same framework. The first question in that Catechism is: "What is the chief end of man?" The answer required is: "To glorify God and to enjoy him forever." Those Calvinists with their heavy theology have been accused of inventing the capitalist system and the Protestant ethic (which is to work hard and save your money). But in their confession of faith, our number one duty is not hard work or good deeds. Rather, according to these divines, our whole purpose is to glorify God, and we do that by enjoying Him. Those early theologians displayed remarkable understanding of our psychological and physical needs.

In John 15:11 Jesus says, "These things I have spoken to you, that my joy may be in you, and that your joy may be full" (RSV). Jesus tells his disciples that his wish for them is a life full of joy and happiness.

If you want to know if this chapter is for you, take this quick test. On a scale of one to ten, rate yourself on how happy you are right at this moment. Ten would represent total happiness, and one none at all. I would say, to start with, that it would be almost impossible to score a one. If you were in that state, you'd be too depressed to be reading a book. By the same token, very few of us are number ten, or at least not consistently. But having set those limitations, what score would you give yourself? If you are an eight or above, this chapter is not likely to be pertinent for you. If you are somewhere between four or seven, it's just possible that you don't have the courage to be happy. And this may be the very thing keeping you from the health and wholeness of body and spirit which God wants to give you.

We've already established that happiness does not depend on circumstances. We can to a large extent make up our minds to be happy—or miserable. I heard a story recently that speaks to this point. A certain man, very much addicted to astrology, consulted his private astrologer every week and tried to follow any instructions. One night he was chatting about these experiences with some friends. His horoscope for the week had been: Make three new friends this week and see what happens. "I did what my astrologer told me," complained the man. "I made three new friends—and nothing happened. Now I'm stuck with three new friends." A lot of us are like that. New friends, a new job, or a new house—none of these are enough. Without the courage to be happy even winning the lottery will probably not do it for us. But those people who have the capacity for happiness or the gift of joy somehow seem to prosper in many ways, not least of all physically. They may, in addition, be joggers, teetotalers, vegetarians, or practitioners of Yoga. But just as many are undisciplined, lazy, overweight, indulging themselves with pasta and gravies, booze, and cigarettes. The irresponsible person full of joy can often be healthier than the stressful, worried person who is a Puritan in diet and habit.

A cheerful heart

Doctors have been telling me for years that "you can't kill a happy man." When I press for an explanation, they suggest that unhappiness often precedes an illness. Happy people rarely get sick and tend to recover quickly when they do get sick. The unhappy person is the target for any and every kind of illness.

In the beginning of this book we talked about Norman Cousins and the healing chronicled in his *Anatomy of An Illness as Perceived by the Patient.* This prestigious literary figure, a layman in the medical world, is now teaching doctors how to practice a different kind of medicine. His schedule is crammed to the hilt and his classes are packed. Laughter was a big part of his self-treatment. He discovered, as we said earlier, that ten minutes of solid belly-laughter would give him two hours of pain-free sleep.

The discovery Cousins made a decade ago, which saved his

life, is now being corroborated by scientists. It seems the brain causes the cells to produce proteins called endoenzymes, which are natural, morphinelike pain-killers. Laughter triggers the production of these endoenzymes. Doctors now agree that Cousin's self-prescribed therapy of joy has a scientific basis. Laughter reduces pain and actually helps to cure the patient. With laughter as his pain-killer, Cousins no longer had to use sleeping pills and other drugs that alter the endocrine system and interfere with the body's own internal healing mechanism.

It's a remarkable story. A brave layman faced with death or immobilizing arthritis finds out something about the nature of healing that is presently at the very forefront of modern medicine. Norman Cousins could find some pertinent texts for his experience in the Old Testament. Jeremiah 46:11 states, "In vain you have used many medicines; there is no healing for you," while Proverbs 17:22 tells us, "A cheerful heart is a good medicine, but a downcast spirit dries up the bones."

Pierre Teilhard de Chardin, a pivotal Christian thinker of our time, said, "Joy is the surest sign of the presence of God." This Jesuit priest-theologian-anthropologist had a good deal in common with the Presbyterian sages who penned the Westminster Confession of Faith. The bottom line for you and me is simply this: grimness is *not* a Christian virtue. There are no sad saints. If God really is the center of one's life and being, joy is inevitable. If we have no joy, we have missed the heart of the Good News and our bodies as much as our souls will suffer the consequences.

Happiness or joy

Let me suggest here a distinction between happiness and joy. I see them as very similar but not quite the same thing. Happiness is the result of being pleased with who we are and what we do, and we can *choose* to have this kind of happiness, whatever the external circumstances. Joy, on the other hand, is the gift that comes from One whom it is perfect joy to know. Joy comes from knowing that the ultimate Person in the universe has chosen us and loved us and forgiven us. We may be old, sick, friendless, poor, blind, halt, and lame. But if we know the Source and Giver of life, we have the gift of joy.

A major obstacle

If we're going to have the courage to be happy, I believe we need to exercise our power to choose, which we have touched on in earlier chapters. The mystery is that often we do choose to live in such unsatisfying ways that we cannot be happy. Why? is a relevant question for any concerned student of the human scene. It seems to me that our need to justify ourselves is one of the biggest obstacles to choosing happiness. We have been saying how difficult it is to admit being wrong and having made mistakes. We think if we do so we will be counted out of the game of life. We spend our whole lives defending ourselves against any possible charge, proving that we have never done wrong or been wrong.

I believe this kind of self-justification is the very heart of sin. God in Jesus Christ has forgiven us and has paid the price for our sins. To claim that forgiveness we must accept the fact that we are wrong; in fact, the Good News is that we are all bad. But we all seem to be so reluctant to acknowledge this. Instead we spend much time and energy getting ourselves off the hook, trying to make ourselves look good or come out smelling like roses.

Perhaps one of the best ways of excusing ourselves from being the persons God wants us to be is to be overworked, overburdened, in a place that is no fun, doing jobs that no one wants to do—in short, living a thankless, unfulfilling sort of existence Then if we fail—as I do frequently—we can say to ourselves or to anyone who will listen, "Well, what do you expect? If you knew how much I had to do and how hard my life is, and how many demands there are on me, you would certainly forgive my failures."

In my early years as a pastor of a small church in the Midwest,

I approached my job in just that way. I was worn out and exhausted at the end of each day. The church was a small one, full of loving people, and no one ever suggested that I should do more. In retrospect, I can remember being told, "Slow down. Don't work so hard. We love you. Don't take life so seriously." Since that time, I've been trying to understand why I did so much. I think it might have been because it gave me a built-in excuse for a possible failure. If my sermon was less than gripping on Sunday morning, I could blame it on a midnight hospital call the night before. I could excuse any chore undone or done poorly, any hostile remark to a parishioner with the fact that I was trying to do the work of two or three men. My own unhappiness was a built-in self-justification mechanism. I preached grace, but I was living by merit. My demanding schedule excused the failures that kept occurring with embarrassing regularity.

In recent years God has been trying to teach me about a new, joyful way to live. Though it sounds selfish, I don't believe it is. It takes real courage, because it has no built-in justification for failure. I am committed to choosing to schedule my time to do those things I really want to do. When I receive an invitation to speak, write or serve on some board, I put it to two tests. First of all do I think it's something God wants me to do? Second, is this something *I* want to do? If I feel positive on both scores, I say yes with enthusiasm. There are other requests that I'm not sure that God is in, even though the person calling may assure me that God has guided him or her to make the request. If, in addition, I don't feel it would be rewarding or interesting or fun to do, I am learning to say no. If joy is the surest sign of the presence of God, and if I have no joy, I work against God's best plan for that situation.

All this has been very difficult for me, mostly because I still need to have everybody like me. I thought if I said no, I would not be liked. I am learning that you are not necessarily liked even when you say yes.

Now or never

A few years ago, someone suggested to me that the parable of the wise and foolish virgins is really about joy. Jesus tells us the virgins are waiting for the bridegroom and each has a lamp—some with oil and some empty. When the bridegroom comes, those who have oil and are ready to light their lamp are invited in to the celebration. Those who have no oil to light their lamps are told the door is closed to them forever. Even though they protest and offer to rush out to the 7-11 to buy some oil, the bridegroom does not relent. It was a case of oil now or never.

I used to think that parable was about preparedness—that we need to be prepared for life's ultimate moment. But the Bible says that the Lord will come as a thief in the night and there will be no time to prepare. I believe our Lord, who was a Jew, was telling this story in terms of His Jewish perspective and background, and in the Old Testament oil almost always represents gladness. As the very symbol of joy, it was an essential part of many spiritual celebrations in those ancient days. The parable indicates to me that joy is not something we can wait to get at some future date. We have joy in the present or not at all.

If joy is a gift from God, not depending upon circumstances, there is no excuse for not having it now. You may think you will have joy when all your ducks are lined up. You'll have joy when you get that unexpected raise, or pay off the mortgage. You'll have it when your kids quit smoking pot and your tennis elbow has healed and your boss quits picking on you. If you're waiting to find joy, this parable suggests you will never have it. You can have it now with all the strange present circumstances of your life.

Paul, in spite of all the harrowing circumstances of his life, had joy. He says, "In whatever state I am, I have learned to be content." He is telling us we can find that which is pleasing in whatever state. There is also much that is unpleasing in whatever state we are. I learned something about this from a

127

There's a lot more to health than not being sick

friend last year. Still unmarried at age twenty-five, he had just quit his job and was leaving with his modest savings to roam the world for a year in search of adventure. He said, "You know, it's tough. I'm really lonely. Most of my colleagues at work are married. They go home every night to someone who cares for them. I go home alone. But, on the other hand, I have a freedom they don't have. Their family responsibilities tie them down to regular jobs. I am free to quit my job and leave on a great adventure. I'm aware that they envy me. I'm coming to understand that the whole secret of life is to enjoy the benefits of your present state without bemoaning the things you don't have. I realize that nobody has it all."

Joy in any state

That young man's philosophy is apropos to all that we're saying in this chapter. There are benefits particular to any age group. There are great benefits to being young. The young usually have health, energy and the prospect of an unlimited future, but most lack position or power or money. There are great benefits to being middle-aged, at the peak of earning powers, creative capacity, and decision-making involvement of all kinds. But accompanying all that are often burdens and responsibilities for the care of younger or older family members. Old age, at best, can bring wisdom, security, and leisure, but also the beginning of physical deterioration. Strength and energy are diminished. The stimulation of the day-to-day challenge in the marketplace is over. I believe the secret of life is to enjoy whichever age we are in without longing for the things we don't have, seizing the moment and the situation and squeezing from it all we can. It is so easy to despair in any condition—youth, middle age or old age. Instead, we can make Paul our model and say with him, "In whatever state I am, I have learned to be content."

Joyful service

A life full of happiness and joy takes great courage and provides very few hiding places. I am no longer the victim of my schedule or demands of others. I choose to do those things which are pleasing to me. I can choose to get enough rest, enough relaxation. When I fail, I have only God's mercy and forgiveness to fall back on.

When we claim God's gift of joy we bless those around us and do away with the tedium of dutiful service. If I have a late-day appointment with my doctor, I hope he won't say to his nurse in a weary voice, "Do you mean there's another patient out there? I suppose I'll have to see him. Send Larson in." I want a doctor who delights in seeing me and who is eager to help me. If I am in the hospital, I don't want a nurse who grumbles that "Larson's ringing his bell again." I hope I'll get a nurse who for some mysterious reason enjoys serving me, giving me a back rub, and even carrying the bedpan. I am blessed by teachers who are excited about the prospect of teaching me, and who bring their joy to the classroom. I want a preacher who can't wait to tell me the Good News every Sunday morning and who thinks that I am an exciting parishioner. Deliver me from the preacher who is weary in well-doing and who is going to tell me one more time to shape up.

I guess I am saying that I don't want to be somebody's project. I don't want to be served out of a sense of duty or even because you love Jesus, and He tells you to care for the last and the least, of which you think I am the most outstanding example. I want the people who teach me, treat me, or serve me in any way to be those people with the courage to be happy.

Our Christian heroes had this gift. St. Francis of Assisi gave up his inheritance to become a servant of lepers, beggars, slaves, pirates, and all the least and the last. He was called *joculator domini*, the "hilarious saint." There was no longsuffering in his arduous life of service. Can you imagine Mother Teresa with her

129

There's a lot more to health than not being sick

alarm going off at 4:00 A.M. in Calcutta getting up and saying, "Oh my, another hard day in this wretched ghetto." I have a feeling she is eager to get up every morning and excited about the prospect of meeting Jesus in a dozen or a hundred new forms as she cares for the sick and the dying.

I often wish I could have visited the late Albert Schweitzer while he was living in Lambaréné in Equatorial Africa. But let's pretend that I did visit him and that one morning crossing the compound I encountered the great man, joined him in a walk, and asked him how things were going. Can you imagine a reply something like this?—"Oh, I'm glad you asked. I have terrible troubles evey morning because of lower back pain. I have a rotten mattress—so lumpy that I can't move around comfortably for hours. And you know that there are holes in my screens and those tsetse flies come in and drive me wild. They keep me awake all night. Have you noticed how bad the food is? Every morning the oatmeal is cold and lumpy and though the cook claims she adds raisins, I think they're flies. After all that, I have to go to surgery where one nurse has BO and the other bad breath."

You and I both know that is *not* what Schweitzer would have said though it's possible that he could have had all of those complaints. Living where he did, it's not inconceivable he suffered from lumpy mattresses, uncertain food, and holes in the screens. But I'd still be willing to bet that on any given morning he was full of joy and enthusiasm about the work there—a nurse coming in from the bush for training, the new wing about to be built, new shipments of medicine to help the patients. When God gives us the gift of joy, He gives us the eyes to see life as it is and the passion to live life risking all for His causes.

I am aware, though, that there are jobs in which there is very little cause for joy. It seems to me that homemakers have a special problem in this area. They serve long hours doing tasks that never get "finished," but they have none of the incentives that operate in the business world like raises and promotions. If

130

you are a homemaker, male or female (and the number of male homemakers is increasing), it is very possible that your spouse does not appreciate your never-ending efforts to keep the house clean, the larder full, and the clothes laundered. Most children take all this service for granted and are not especially grateful. An awful lot of overworked homemakers living with unappreciative families end up full of longsuffering and joylessness.

If you happen to be one of the homemakers that I just described, I suggest you cease doing those household chores at the point where they begin to be burdensome. Work as long as it feels good. When it ceases to feel good, stop and do something that will rekindle your own happiness. Indulge yourself in something that you consider fun or which has meaning for you. You may sit down and read a book. You may visit a friend. You may start meeting with a small group for Bible study. You may start visiting at the hospital. You may play some tennis or take up a new and creative hobby. You may start working on that long delayed novel you always intended to write.

That may mean that the shirts won't be ironed that day. It may mean scrapping the plans for a gourmet meal and simply opening some cans or serving sandwiches. But when your family begins to dribble in the front door, they're going to be greeted with enthusiasm by a person full of joy instead of by the usual overworked, drudge. The gift of joy beats gourmet meals and vacuumed rugs and polished furniture and will knock their socks off, as none of that service ever did. You might change the whole climate of your household. By "selfishly" taking care of your own needs, you can be a blessing to the people around you.

The same kind of counsel can apply to any of us—students, factory workers, business or professional people. To have your life full of more tasks than you can possibly finish will rob you of joy and happiness, and that will affect those with whom you live and work. How much we need to find those things that are essential to do and then zero in on those. In other words, we need to simplify our lives.

There's a lot more to health than not being sick

Finding the essentials

On an early spring day in Washington, D.C., a new excursion boat was making its way up the Potomac on its maiden run. To inaugurate this event, a large number of Congressmen and senators had been invited, along with some members of the press. The sun was bright and hot, and one famous senator had removed his shoes and socks and settled back in a deck chair to wiggle his toes. The socks were hung on a railing in front of him.

One of the columnists aboard was observing all this when someone running along the deck inadvertently brushed against one of the socks. It fell over the railing into the river and was quickly swallowed in the wake of the ship. The columnist was particularly impressed by what followed next, and it confirmed in his mind this legislator's true genius. The senator, seeing what had happened, calmly went over to the railing, picked up his remaining sock and threw it overboard. Writing about the incident later, the columnist confessed that if the same thing had happened to him, he would have taken the one remaining sock and put it in his pocket and brought it home. "I have a whole drawerful of single socks at home. I won't ever find the mate, but one cannot throw away a perfectly good single sock. My life is full of single socks. Things that have no possible use for me. There is so much in my life like that but I realize that I've got to clean out all the things that are perfectly good, but good for nothing, and get down to some simple basics."

Even if our lives are full of only good and useful things, there can be too many of them and they can cause us to end up harried and worried and overworked. We've gotten into that predicament by choice and we can choose to get out of it. Remember, it takes great courage to be happy, and that may mean throwing out our single socks, simplifying our lives, and doing less of those things that ultimately help no one. It means finding those exciting and meaningful things and doing them with gusto.

9.

Guidelines and conclusions about wellness

"Within the last several years, there has been a growing realization of what many of us had known all along, that emotional caring can be as important to the patient's overall health and well-being as physical curing."

—*Irene Kraus*, The Importance of Caring

Every week I come upon new insights into the nature ϳf ϣɑn and the spiritual implications of health. The door to the future is swinging wider and wider and we see increasingly through the eyes of doctors, psychiatrists and psychologists what it means to be a whole person.

I'm reluctant to write this concluding chapter because I anticipate that a new discovery tomorrow will throw even more light on the causes of illness and the positive approaches to health. The concept of wellness, though fairly new, is dynamic, and the medical profession is having a hard time keeping up, let alone average lay people. More and more writers and speakers are discussing wellness. Bits and pieces of information on the subject keep surfacing—arriving in the mail or being featured on the front page of our newspapers' science section or on our favorite television talk shows.

Researchers and proponents of wellness agree on some of its ingredients—things like good nutrition and adequate rest. Beyond that, however, they name more nebulous qualities such as feeling good about yourself, coping with conflicts and stress, having concrete life goals and purposes. One such proponent of wellness is John Pilch of Milwaukee, a sort of twentieth century John the Baptist whose prophetic lectures emphasize the correlation of spiritual values to wellness. He has said, "The key elements of wellness are knowing the purpose of life, understanding its genuine joys and pleasures and assuming total and complete self-responsibility."

Curing our own ills

Breakthroughs in drugs and medicines continue to reinforce this new thrust. Most of us have been reading about the discovery of a substance called interferon. Interferon seems to be the miracle drug we have all been looking for, a cure for all kinds of diseases from the common cold to cancer. It is not being widely used at present simply because it is so expensive to manufacture. Until very recently, the human body was the only source of interferon. Think about it. The human body has the capacity for manufacturing this miracle drug, but the problem is that the body does not seem to produce sufficient quantities at the appropriate times. Right now the experts are looking for less costly ways to produce synthetic interferon. I wish them success, but I would rather see us working toward increasing the release of our natural interferon through the practice of positive attitudes, spiritual values, or disciplines of the mind. If this miracle substance could be manufactured by our bodies in larger quantities and released as needed, we would have the power to cure most of our own ills. It boggles the mind to learn that the power to heal, whether it is the common cold or cancer, lies locked within the mystery of the human body itself.

The power of faith

Recently one of my new parishioners stopped by my office to report on a medical convention she had attended in Boston. She teaches medicine, and she was excited about a report made at the convention by Dr. Barry Wyke of London, a member of the Royal College of Surgeons. He had presented documented proof that physical changes occur in the body when people *believe* they're going to be well. This doctor is a devout atheist and a hard-nosed scientist whose research is available in the University of Massachusetts Medical School Library and the Medical Line Computer. Certainly his idea is not new for those of us who are Christians; the New Testament is full of stories of miraculous healings: the lame walked, the blind saw, the mentally disturbed were restored to sanity, simply because they believed in Jesus and His power to heal. The body responded to the word of faith and hope and love, and miraculous cures took place.

Another doctor who seems to take a nonmedical approach to health is Dr. Raymond Moody, Jr. Like Norman Cousins, Dr. Moody reports on the therapeutic benefits of laughter. His new book, *Laugh After Laugh: The Healing Power of Humor*, is full of scholarly research and whimsical insight and provides historical examples, scientific hypotheses, and modern case studies to support his thesis: namely, that the kind of good humor which is one part hope and one part hilarity is a tremendous asset to personal health.

Another exciting book that deals with the spiritual dimensions of health is Dr. William A. Nolen's *A Surgeon's Book of Hope*. Dr. Nolen, who is chief of surgery at Meeker County Hospital in Litchfield, Minnesota, emphasizes in his book the "mysterious will to live" that astounds the medical world and is almost *the* most important factor in the prevention and cure of illness. This book about hope gives us hope—hope for the whole medical world. Dr. Nolen warns against absolutism in medicine: "The most unforgivable inadequacy of the doctor as a human being, is when, by attitude and diminishing interest, he places distance between himself and the patient he has concluded is hopeless." Dr. Nolen understands the mysterious healing power of relationships. Medicine may be a science, but the art of healing is a gift. My hope and belief is that his tribe in medicine will increase in the coming decade.

A dual affair

Norman Cousins had this to say about the doctor-patient relationship in the August 1980 *Saturday Review:* "The physician's job is to bring to the encounter [with the patient] the best that medical science has to offer. The patient brings a healing system that can be activated by a strong will to live, powerful expectations of recovery and a sense of control over his or her autonomic nervous system. Conversely, feelings of panic can retard the healing process by impairing the ability of the human brain to produce the secretions that are essential to recovery. The wise physician recognizes that his job is not just to administer medication but to engage the emotional resources of the patient to the fullest. This is what is meant by the physician-patient partnership."

I read about a doctor in Denver who is practicing this new kind of physician-patient relationship. His patient had cancer of the prostate which had metastasized to the skull, hips, spine— 250 lesions altogether. Medically speaking, the man had at most four weeks to live. His doctor told him, "If you believe this cancer is terminal, it will be. You and I will go into a partnership. I'll give you everything medicine knows—surgery, estrogen, whatever is needed. I want *you* to have the best time of your life: laugh, do what you want to do, begin to see it as funny." Today that man is still alive, the lesions have mostly cleared, and somebody from the Stanford Medical School is writing up the case.

Deadly emotions

The evidence that our positive emotions—hope, laughter, and the like—can make us well is piling up. Just as inescapable, though, is the evidence that our negative emotions are making us sick. In the September 1980 issue of *Psychology Today*, Maggie Scarf writes about Dr. Carl Simonton and his psychologist wife Stefanie Matthews-Simonton and their treatment of cancer types. "The Simontons argue there is a cancer-prone personality, that certain combinations of traits make some people especially vulnerable to cancer. Simonton listed these characteristics in a 1975 article: 'First, a great tendency to hold resentment and marked inability to forgive; second, a tendency to self-pity; third, a poor ability to develop and maintain meaningful long-term relationships; and fourth, a very poor self-image.' These qualities, Simonton proposes, make it difficult for a person to deal with emotions at a conscious level, to acknowledge negative feelings and then to deal with them. The feelings which the Simontons term 'negative emotions' . . . are eventually given somatic expression. Malignancy is thus despair that has been experienced biologically, despair at the level of the cell."

If the Simonton research has validity, then it does not take a great stretch of the imagination to realize the role that Christian faith can play in healing this kind of emotionally rooted illness. Faith leads to hope which leads to love which transforms personalities and grounds us in the security of God's love and acceptance. In this climate or ambience it is O.K. to express negative feelings.

A new kind of hospital

There are even some hospitals reorganizing their agendas so that they can minister to the emotional needs as well as the physical needs of the patients. Irene Kraus, chairman of the American Hospital Association, has written a book entitled *The Importance of Caring*. In it she says, "Compassionate, personalized care has long remained the ultimate goal of hospitals. In fact, in the early days of hospitals and medicines, caring was often a sole aid that physicians and nurses could give to their patients. Many diseases had no cure; medical capabilities to relieve suffering were limited. Because cures were not possible, caring was the only alternative.

"Within the last several years, there has been a growing realization of what many of us had known all along, that emotional caring can be as important to the patient's overall health and well-being as physical curing."

She goes on to say, "The principles of compassion and helpful care are based in part on the spiritual values of religions and in part on the moral values important in the philosophy of a democratic nation. Both principles proclaim the inherent value and dignity of each man. So all hospitals, not just religion-based institutions, are responsible to their community for humanistic care.

"The development of a truly caring hospital begins with people who work in them. We cannot assume that the responsibility for humanistic care belongs solely to employees; it is the responsibility of the community and the administration as well."

Those of us who have ever been in a hospital can cheer for Irene Kraus and her worthy goal. Too many of us have been victims of impersonal, inadequate, and incompetent care in medical institutions. Irene Kraus not only sees the need for compassionate, personalized care; she understands that only people with deep spiritual values are motivated to provide that kind of care. More than that, she sees the community itself and the hospital staff as partners in this kind of care.

Predicting illness

One of the oldest research projects exploring the relationship between mind, spirit, and body has been going on for the past thirty-eight years among a group of men who were college sophomores in an Eastern university in the 1940s. Investigators have been making periodic checks on the physical and mental health of this group. Their findings indicate that poor mental health is a key predicter of early physical deterioration, according to Dr. George Valliant of the psychiatry department at Cambridge Hospital in Cambridge, Massachusetts. Of forty-eight men who had the worst mental health between the ages of twenty-one and forty-six, eighteen were hit with chronic illness or death by the age of fifty-three.

"This isn't a question of bad health affecting happiness or adjustment," explains Valliant, "because our work shows that

140

these men were badly adjusted well before their health started to deteriorate." The most startling part of the study was that alcohol and tobacco use, obesity and the life-span of parents and grandparents were not the determining factors in health and longevity that we have been assuming. While these factors did have some effect on the men's physical well-being, their mental health seemed to predetermine their physical well-being independently of whether they smoked, drank, were overweight or had parents who died young. In other words, men in robust health at fifty-three weren't necessarily those whose parents had lived to a ripe old age and who had practiced good health habits themselves. Emotional problems eventually produced physical illness in spite of disciplined living and good genes. Valliant cautions, "I'm not recommending that people smoke or let themselves get overweight!" Certainly habits and genes do affect health to a large degree, but mental attitude plays a powerful role in what happens to our bodies. Valliant concludes, "No matter what, the men who were better at loving, who had more satisfying personal relations, seem to avoid early aging, while the health of poor emotional copers was significantly more likely to deteriorate during middle age."

What can I do?

Health is still a mystery that eludes us. We all know people who are pronounced fit at their annual checkup by medical experts and then drop dead within the week. In addition, we all know people who break all the rules of good health and yet seem to live forever and remain well. Having said that, what is the reasonable and sound approach to the whole matter of our own wellness? I would suggest at least five things:

1. If you have some physical symptoms indicating a health problem, by all means see a *good* doctor. I say a good doctor, for we all know there are many kinds of doctors. Find one who knows the science of medicine and practices the art of healing. Have yourself checked out physically. If surgery or radical

treatment is recommended, get a second opinion and possibly even a third. Don't be timid about this. No one is an expert in the area of *your* body and *your* health.

2. The genes you have inherited are an important clue to your health and longevity, but they don't necessarily determine your future well-being. Good genes from healthy parents who lived a long time are a great legacy. But one can fall victim to illness or premature death even with good genes. On the other hand, one can inherit bad genes and overcome them. A doctor who treated me for years had lost both of his parents while they were in their forties. This pattern frightened him enough to make radical changes in his own lifestyle. Already a profound Christian, he became an avid jogger and a vegetarian. At age fifty-five he shows no signs of deteriorating.

3. Man is more spiritual than physical. Our bodies are barometers of our inner, nontangible experiences, thoughts, fears, angers, resentments, hopes, joys. It is safe to say that 90 percent of most physical ailments have a real emotional, spiritual connection. Don't ignore the physical but be aware that attitudes, feelings and emotions are perhaps even more important. Honor the fact that your body is the barometer that registers the condition of your spiritual life.

4. Believe that God designed your body to resist illness. One must really work hard to become ill and stay ill. The body's natural illness-resistance makes it difficult to get sick. Illness can be a sign that something is wrong in your life, in your lifestyle, your relationships, etc. Remember that there are healing forces within each of us to combat any form of illness that finally overtakes us. The body is capable of producing the very substances that effect most cures.

5. Health is more than non-illness. The best medical, psychiatric and psychological knowledge we have today indicates that wellness or wholeness is far more than not being ill. If a doctor could cure every disease in your body, you still might not be well and might not be everything you were meant to be. But if you are striving for wholeness, the odds are that you will have

minimal illness. In other words, while nonillness cannot be equated with health, those who have personal wholeness have minimized their chances of getting ill or staying ill.

A model for wholeness

I hope that this book has given you some clues about what it means to be a whole person. By exploring patterns, attitudes, and behaviors that contribute to wellness and wholeness, I have tried to show that there's more to health than not being sick. Much can be learned by looking at the medical and psychological aspects of wholeness and of course, ultimately, from the insights of the Bible. But most of us learn more from models than we do from reading or hearing.

One of my new neighbors in Seattle is an 87-year-old lady who lives a few miles west of me in the Olympic Mountains, in the Hoh River Valley in Jefferson County. Her name is Lena Fletcher and she is the daughter of John Huelsdonk, one of the pioneers of this whole area. Describing her father, who was called "The Iron Man of the Hoh," Mrs. Fletcher says, "Dad wasn't especially tall, but he weighed 240 pounds—all muscle—and he regularly backpacked 130–140 pounds in the woods."

There are many legends about Huelsdonk, who roamed the mountains, glaciers, and forests of Olympic National Park long before it was a park. One reports that a woodsman saw him walking across a log carrying a cast-iron stove on his back. Huelsdonk was transporting this up into the woods for the rangers who were building cabins. The woodsman remarked that the burden looked awfully heavy. Huelsdonk supposedly replied, "The stove isn't bad, but that darn hundred-pound sack of flour in the oven keeps shifting around."

Lena Fletcher, a powerfully built, white-haired lady, works daily in her garden, weeding rows of corn, beans, peas, dill, cucumbers, and rutabagas in the rich river-bottom land. "Other people jog to keep fit," she said. "I work in the garden and split and pile wood. It makes a lot more sense to have something to show for the energy you expend." In her lifetime, Mrs. Fletcher has done postgraduate work; she's been a teacher, a justice of the peace for the western half of Jefferson County, and an active agitator for good government, sound ecology, and good grammar. I marvel at her ability to discourse with faultless memory on such varied subjects as constitutional law, rainfall, wildlife, and the exploits of her father.

This incredible neighbor gives me great hope. She is living life to the full and is in radiant health. One day Lena Fletcher will die. But I don't believe she will ever be old. She is what wellness and wholeness are all about. We're all going to die. Someone has said God plans to get us all in the end. But I believe death is God's good gift to us. Illness and infirmity in old age, on the other hand, are not His intentional will. In this book we have been saying, above all, that we have more autonomy than we think in this whole matter of wellness and wholeness. I covet for each of you readers that you begin to be and do those things that make for health. God is on your side.